Pediatric Patient Safety
in the Emergency Department

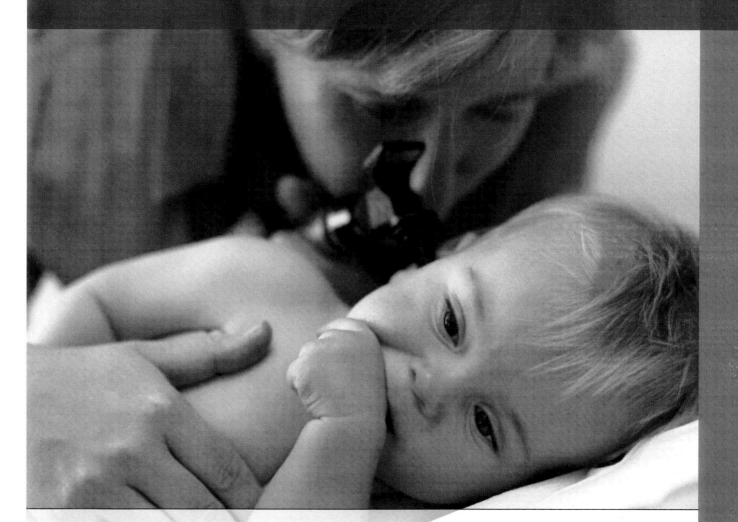

Joint Commission Resources

American Academy
of Pediatrics
DEDICATED TO THE HEALTH OF ALL CHILDREN™

EDITED BY
STEVEN E. KRUG, M.D., F.A.A.P.

FOREWORDS BY
KAREN S. FRUSH, B.S.N., M.D.,
F.A.A.P.
EDWARD S. OGATA, M.D., F.A.A.P.

Editor and Manager, Publications: Victoria Gaudette
Project Manager: Meghan Anderson
Associate Director, Production: Johanna Harris
Executive Director: Catherine Chopp Hinckley, Ph.D.
Joint Commission/JCR Reviewers: Nanne Finis, Mary Lacher, Jeannell Mansur, Richard Molteni, Deborah Nadzam, Francine Westergaard, and Tony Woodward

Joint Commission Resources Mission

The mission of Joint Commission Resources (JCR) is to continuously improve the safety and quality of health care in the United States and in the international community through the provision of education, publications, consultation, and evaluation services.

Joint Commission Resources educational programs and publications support, but are separate from, the accreditation activities of The Joint Commission. Attendees at Joint Commission Resources educational programs and purchasers of Joint Commission Resources publications receive no special consideration or treatment in, or confidential information about, the accreditation process.

The inclusion of an organization name, product, or service in a Joint Commission Resources publication should not be construed as an endorsement of such organization, product, or service, nor is failure to include an organization name, product, or service to be construed as disapproval.

This publication is designed to provide accurate and authoritative information in regard to the subject matter covered. Every attempt has been made to ensure accuracy at the time of publication; however, please note that laws, regulations, and standards are subject to change. Please also note that some of the examples in this publication are specific to the laws and regulations of the locality of the facility. The information and examples in this publication are provided with the understanding that the publisher is not engaged in providing medical, legal, or other professional advice. If any such assistance is desired, the services of a competent professional person should be sought.

Printed in the U.S.A. 5 4 3 2 1

Requests for permission to make copies of any part of this work should be mailed to
Permissions Editor
Department of Publications
Joint Commission Resources
One Renaissance Boulevard
Oakbrook Terrace, Illinois 60181 U.S.A.
permissions@jcrinc.com

ISBN: 978-1-59940-212-3
Library of Congress Control Number: 2009942794

For more information about Joint Commission Resources, please visit http://www.jcrinc.com.

Table of Contents

Foreword by
Edward S. Ogata, M.D., F.A.A.P.

At some point in our lives, most of us will be a patient in a hospital emergency department. Because acute illnesses and injuries of children are always anxiety provoking to parents, children are even more likely to be brought to emergency departments. There they often are placed at risk. They enter an environment that is usually chaotic as the emergency department faces the ongoing challenges of suddenly arriving, acutely ill patients and the pressures of providing care to a large number of awaiting patients, some of whom may have hidden serious disorders. Medical evaluation and transfers tend to be hurried, and handoffs can be limited or inaccurate. In addition, emergency departments in most general hospitals do not have pediatric services sufficiently comprehensive to meet all the needs of children.

To address these challenges, Joint Commission Resources and the American Academy of Pediatrics with Steven Krug, M.D., a senior leader in Pediatric Emergency Medicine, have gathered experts to provide a road map to assure safe care for children in hospital emergency departments. These experts provide guidance to reduce the risks of both active and latent errors. This advice is of great importance to all who work so hard to provide care in the nation's emergency departments.

Edward S. Ogata, M.D., F.A.A.P.
Chief Medical Officer
Northwestern University Feinberg School of Medicine
Children's Memorial Hospital, Chicago

Foreword by Karen S. Frush, B.S.N., M.D., F.A.A.P.

When I walked into the emergency department (ED) one Sunday morning, a resident greeted me with a worried look on his face. "Dr. Frush, we have a problem." He went on to describe an infant who had been cared for in the ED through the night. The young child required treatment with antibiotics after having been brought in by her parents because of a high fever. It had been a very hectic night; the team was short-staffed, a new nurse was being oriented, the resident was working his third straight night shift and it was four o'clock in the morning. As he described later, he was exhausted and felt like he was "hitting the wall." There was no computerized order entry system, so the resident calculated a dose of an appropriate antibiotic for the child and wrote an order. Before the nurse drew up the medicine she checked his math and got the same (wrong) answer. The infant received 10 times the proper dose of the antibiotic, and the day team had just discovered the error as I was arriving in the ED. I was now the "attending of record," and it was my responsibility to share this news with the worried parents who had been pacing at their child's bedside through the night.

One of the most difficult jobs I have as a patient safety leader and a pediatric emergency physician is to disclose medical errors to patients, parents, and families. It's often a devastating experience; clinicians who have often practiced for years and are vigilant, hard-working, dedicated, and well-intentioned individuals suffer greatly when an error occurs and a child is harmed. Yet this suffering pales in comparison to the anguish endured by parents and families of children who die as a result of a medical error. Amazingly, some parents have been able to turn their family tragedies into powerful motivational messages and programs that help clinicians improve patient safety, and prevent harmful events from occurring to any more children. Sorrel King is one example. After her daughter Josie died as a result of a medical error, she established the Josie King Foundation to "prevent others from dying or being harmed by medical errors. By uniting healthcare providers and consumers, and funding innovative safety programs, we hope to create a culture of patient safety, together."

Sorrel recently participated on an expert panel at a national meeting of emergency care professionals, drug manufacturers, pharmacists, representatives from government agencies and others who had gathered to develop solutions for safe delivery of pediatric medications, with a focus on children in the emergency setting. National leaders described a number of problems and inherent risks in the highly complex pediatric medication process. Due to a lack of standard pediatric drug formulations, for example, clinicians are forced to calculate individual drug doses for each pediatric patient. Many EDs in our country still lack computerized order entry systems that provide pre-calculated doses, and even those with advanced IT systems have few pre-determined medication doses that are immediately available to clinicians at the bedside in the setting of a life-threatening emergency. Sorrel was dismayed to learn about the inherent risks in the current system, and she implored us to "fix it" so that we can prevent harm to more children. She also reminded us that although advanced technology is important, communication is a true key to safe care. Effective communication requires that we include patients and families when we develop our plans of care; that we really listen to families so that we can hear their concerns; and that we disclose information related to adverse events in a transparent manner in order to maintain a trusting relationship. As Sorrel summarized her remarks, she challenged all of us who were present at the meeting to "figure it out—please figure out all the answers. Please do everything you can to make care safer for children."

I believe this book is an important part of a larger national effort that is underway to "do everything we can to make emergency care safer for children." Created through the collaborative work of the American Academy of Pediatrics and Joint Commission Resources (JCR), the educational arm of the Joint Commission (TJC), *Pediatric Patient Safety in the Emergency Department* addresses important topics in pediatric patient safety from the perspective of clinicians who provide front-line care for children in individual EDs (microsystems), and from the broad, systems-based perspective of pediatric healthcare leaders, regulators and educators. The authors describe many different activities and programs that have initiated to "fix the problem" and reduce risk in the pediatric emergency care system. Included are examples of safety improvements and best practices from individual hospitals and institutions (such as safety walkrounds, training to improve teamwork and communication, and tools to improve handoffs and transitions in care), as well as recommendations from large multi-disciplinary healthcare professions groups, such as strategies to decrease the risk of radiation exposure for children undergoing radiographic studies, and guidelines

for ED leaders to improve pediatric preparedness. By adopting and implementing these best practices, hospitals and healthcare professionals can achieve safer care and make meaningful changes that will support long-lasting improvements in caring for children in the ED.

This book would not be possible without the leadership, commitment and vision of Steve Krug, M.D., F.A.A.P., who is a champion for pediatric patient safety in the emergency department. Not only has he led changes to improve the safety of children who receive care in the ED where he works, but he has also spent countless hours chairing national committees, leading child advocacy efforts, sharing lessons learned and encouraging colleagues to join the movement to advance patient safety. I hope you'll join this movement, too, as we continue to do all that we possibly can to make emergency care safer for children.

Karen S. Frush, B.S.N., M.D., F.A.A.P.
Chief Patient Safety Officer
Duke University Health System

Preface by Steven E. Krug, M.D., F.A.A.P.

While the Institute of Medicine may have used the word "uneven" in describing the status of pediatric emergency care in the 2006 report, *Emergency Care for Children: Growing Pains,* I prefer to use the analogy of the "perfect storm." The perfect storm is a massive storm, created by the confluence of more than one weather disturbance, creating a substantially more devastating storm. The contributing weather disturbances in the case of pediatric patient safety in the emergency department (ED) are the following:

- Baseline care quality and patient safety concerns that reside in our existing health care systems

- Patient safety issues that reside in all emergency departments, due to the nature of the environment, typically with numerous competing demands for care providers, high patient acuity, multiple interruptions, language barriers, etc.

- The deleterious influence of overcrowding, which now affects nearly every ED in the United States, further magnifying many of the factors noted above

- The unique characteristics and care needs for children, such as weight-based medication dosing, which further increase the risk for medical errors and adverse events

- Deficiencies in day-to-day readiness in many EDs, such as the absence of equipment for children of all ages and sizes, and the level of experience and/or competency of many emergency care providers in the care of children

This is not to suggest that hospitals or ED care providers are negligent in their efforts to care for children. For many, the 4th and 5th bullets reflect the reality of emergency care in the majority of our nation's EDs. While children represent approximately 20 to 25 percent of all ED visits nationwide, there exists a relative "pediatric experience gap" for care providers in the majority of EDs. Ninety percent of children receive their care in a non-children's hospital-based

ED, yet 50% of U.S. EDs care for less than 10 children per day. As the majority of children seeking emergency care are thankfully not severely ill or injured, the on going experience in the assessment and management of very ill or critically injured children for the clinical staff in these EDs is limited. Even for the relative minority of general ED staff that endeavor to obtain and maintain certification in available pediatric emergency or resuscitation courses (e.g., PALS, APLS, ENPC), it is clear that the knowledge and skills obtained during such courses extinguishes quickly.

So, how do hospitals, clinical managers, and front-line staff navigate this perfect storm? Well, the first step is recognizing the presence of a problem, the experience gap, and opportunities to improve pediatric care quality and patient safety. The second step is making the commitment to improve pediatric emergency care, and in doing so, elevating the emergency care needs of children to the level of institutional priority that will result in the allocation of time and necessary resources to close the gap. As recommended in the 2009 joint policy statement, *Guidelines for the Care of Children in the Emergency Department,* published by the American Academy of Pediatrics (AAP), the American College of Emergency Physicians (ACEP), and the Emergency Nurses Association (ENA), this effort to improve emergency readiness for children of all ages is likely to be successful if it is lead by a physician and nurse coordinator for pediatric emergency care. Performance improvement in pediatric care quality, and the reduction of pediatric patient safety concerns, should be pursued bi-directionally, both 'top-down' from hospital leadership and ED managers, as well as 'bottom-up' from front-line staff, who are uniquely positioned to identify and resolve safety concerns. The promotion of a "just culture" by an organization's leadership and ED clinical managers will certainly facilitate this and other patient safety initiatives.

The progress made by a health care organization will be assisted with an awareness of resources such as the AAP/ACEP/ENA policy statement, evidence-based and/or expert consensus driven guidelines and clinical-decision rules, and the growing number of pediatric emergency care resources. In the spirit of adding further to the available resource base for hospital organizations and the thousands of professionals who staff EDs and endeavor to do their best in serving the needs of children and families, the American Academy of Pediatrics and Joint Commission Resources (JCR) have partnered to develop this book, which we hope will provide a sensible and safe path for the many who must navigate this perfect storm.

This book would not be possible without the steadfast commitment of the leadership of both the AAP and JCR to improve pediatric care quality and safety in the ED setting and their desire to partner in this project. Likewise, this resource would not be possible without the outstanding contributions of many patient safety and pediatric care experts from JCR and AAP. Finally, the consistently

professional support from AAP and JCR staff was an essential factor toward the completion of a high quality resource. I would also be remiss if I did not acknowledge the influence of the many who continue to inspire me (my family, my division colleagues and our ED staff at Children's Memorial Hospital, the many trainees I have been fortunate to teach [or to learn from], my pediatric emergency medicine colleagues nationwide, and the many children and families I have been privileged to care for) to continue to improve what I do and to do what I can to help/teach/inspire others to do the same. Carpe diem!

Steven E. Krug, M.D., F.A.A.P.
Head, Division of Emergency Medicine
Children's Memorial Hospital, Chicago, Illinois
Professor of Pediatrics, Northwestern
University Feinberg School of Medicine
Past-Chair, AAP Committee on
Pediatric Emergency Medicine
Chair, AAP Disaster Preparedness Advisory Council

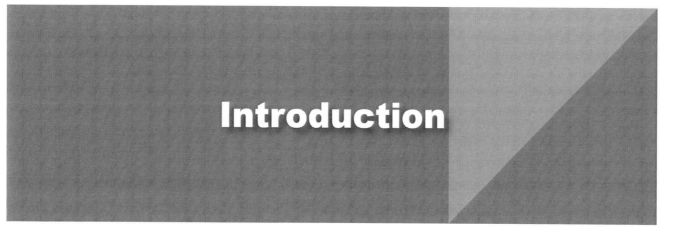

Introduction

Emergency departments (EDs) provide a vital service to the communities they serve as a source of life saving care for patients in need. The ED is also an essential component of a health care safety net, particularly for the many patients—including children—who face barriers in efforts to access care through a medical home. As children represent a significant percentage (20%) of patients seeking emergency care,[1] pediatric preparedness in the ED is essential for delivering appropriate and safe care to ill and injured children.

Caring for children in the ED can be quite challenging and is prone to safety concerns due to a number of environmental and human factors.[2] The ED setting is often hectic and chaotic, with frequent workflow interruptions and barriers to effective communication. Most children in the United States—nearly 90%—are cared for in EDs that are located in general hospitals rather than in hospitals dedicated to the care of children.[1,3] Because a minority of patients in general hospitals are in the pediatric age group, many ED staff may lack familiarity with pediatric emergencies and sufficient opportunities to regularly practice the cognitive and technical skills, such as medication administration, necessary for providing pediatric emergency care.[2]

The Institute of Medicine (IOM) has noted that many hospital EDs are not equally capable of caring for children and adults, and that the needs of children, at times, have been overlooked.[4,5] The 2006 IOM report, "Emergency Care for Children: Growing Pains", noted the continued presence of significant deficiencies, including insufficient pediatric emergency care training and continuing professional education for ED staff, and the absence of key pediatric equipment and medications in many EDs.[5] As the majority of EDs in the United States care for less than 10 children per day, the IOM and others have acknowledged the presence of great variability in the on-going pediatric clinical experience for many hospital-based emergency care providers.[2,3,5]

In a recent study evaluating clinical performance during mock drills conducted in 35 EDs in North Carolina, including 5 trauma centers, nearly all of the EDs in the study committed significant errors in their efforts to stabilize seriously injured children during trauma simulations.[6] Although all EDs strive to give the highest quality of care to patients no matter what their age, research suggests that a lack of pediatric patient readiness is not unique to EDs in North Carolina.[3,4] Studies have demonstrated that many EDs may not maintain the full range of equipment necessary to care for children of all ages, and that ED leaders are unaware of published guidelines for pediatric emergency care.[3,5,7]

Responding to the need to enhance the day-to-day pediatric readiness of EDs and the quality and safety of emergency care provided to children, the American Academy of Pediatrics, the American College of Emergency Physicians, the Emergency Nurses Association, along with a number of endorsing professional organizations, have published a joint policy statement, *Guidelines for Care of Children in the Emergency Department,* that specifies the critical components necessary for optimal emergency care for children of all ages.[8] This policy statement identifies necessary ED leadership; equipment, medication and supplies; physician and nurse qualifications; quality improvement and patient safety guidelines; policies, procedures and protocols; and support services that should be in place in every ED. These recommendations, published in October 2009, offer insight into the components necessary for optimal pediatric emergency care and stress the importance that these elements relate to one another to form a more comprehensive and effective pediatric care delivery system.

Is your ED optimally prepared for pediatric patients?

A Collaboration Between Joint Commission Resources and the American Academy of Pediatrics

Pediatric patient safety spans the missions of Joint Commission Resources (JCR) and the American Academy of Pediatrics (AAP), which is why these organizations have come together to create *Pediatric Patient Safety in the Emergency Department.*

Designed to help leaders of hospitals and emergency care centers to understand pediatric care needs, integrate the necessary resources, and sustain successful practices to improve the emergency care they provide to children, this book and CD feature discussions, strategies, and tips that focus on the unique needs and concerns of caring for pediatric patients. Reviewed, edited, and authored by experts from AAP and JCR, each chapter focuses on a critical component of caring for pediatric patients in the ED. Chapter topics include:

- Hospital leadership and its impact on pediatric care in the ED
- Communication involving pediatric patients and their families in the ED and beyond
- Promoting a patient and family-centered Environment of Care® in the ED
- Medication safety for pediatric patients in the ED
- Infection prevention and control issues unique to pediatric patients in the ED
- Pediatric patient assessment, diagnostic studies, and treatment in the ED
- Treating children with special health care needs in the ED
- Including pediatric care needs in disaster management

Overview of the Book

Chapter 1, "Hospital Leadership and Its Impact on Pediatric Care in the ED," edited by Richard A. Molteni, M.D., F.A.A.P., and Steven E. Krug, M.D., F.A.A.P., discusses the vital role hospital leadership plays to ensure its emergency department is prepared for pediatric patients. Chapter topics include the following:

- Emergency medical services for children
- The front door of the hospital organization
- The essential role for pediatric care leadership and advocacy in the ED
- Forming a LILY team
- Planning and budgeting for pediatric care

- Emphasizing training and continuing education in pediatric care
- Partnering with the community and building awareness
- Adhering to leadership standards and guidelines

Chapter 2, "Communication Involving Pediatric Patients and Their Families in the ED and Beyond," edited by Tony Woodward, M.D., M.B.A., F.A.A.P., addresses the essential need for clear and effective communication throughout an organization, and specifically focuses on:

- Encouraging communication between ED professionals
- Strengthening initial (pre-admission or pre-arrival) communication
- Gaining the trust of patients and families

Chapter 3, "Promoting a Patient and Family-Centered Environment of Care® in the ED," edited by Francine Westergaard, R.N., M.S.N., M.B.A., stresses why organizations should strive to create a patient and family-centered environment of care and features discussions on the following:

- Adopting family-centered care in the ED
- Supporting family presence during all aspects of care
- Providing comfort for children in distress
- The collaborative health care team
- Improving pediatric patient safety in the ED

Chapter 4, "Medication Safety for Pediatric Patients in the ED," authored by Jeannell Mansur, Pharm.D., F.A.S.H.P., offers key information on ways to ensure that ED medication safety policies and practices address the specific needs of pediatric patients. The chapter focuses on the following:

- Medication reconciliation
- Medication safety in the ED: addressing the fundamentals
- Requirements for labeling medications
- Safe medication prescribing for children in the ED
- Relying on pharmacists in the medication use process
- Using technology to enhance pediatric medication safety
- Prescribing home-going medications from the ED
- Monitoring and managing pediatric sedation and analgesia
- Pain management

Chapter 5, "Infection Prevention and Control Issues Unique to Pediatric Patient in the ED," authored by Andrea T. Cruz, M.D., M.P.H., F.A.A.P., and Coburn H.

Allen, M.D., F.A.A.P., addresses infection prevention and control issues specific to pediatric patients and focuses on the following:

- General principles of infection control
- Surveillance
- Bioterrorism
- Pandemic influenza
- Specific infection control scenarios

Chapter 6, "Pediatric Patient Assessment, Diagnostic Studies, and Treatment in the ED," authored by Steven E. Krug, M.D., F.A.A.P., discusses what EDs can do to ensure they are prepared to assess, diagnose, and treat children. The following topics are included:

- Customizing the emergency care process for children
- Determining when to proceed with diagnostic testing
- Developing emergency care practices that involve patient families
- Assessing the risks and benefits of medical imaging for children
- Being prepared for pediatric trauma
- Anticipating the interfacility transfer of pediatric patients
- Maintaining vigilance for non-accidental trauma and child maltreatment
- Mental health emergencies in children and adolescents
- Adopting an evidence-based approach to pediatric emergency care

Chapter 7, "Treating Children with Special Health Care Needs in the ED," edited by Loren G. Yamamoto, M.D., M.P.H., F.A.A.P., outlines issues specific to caring for children with special health care needs and offers discussions on:

- Understanding the unique issues in caring for children with special health care needs
- Supporting care coordination
- Managing devices and equipment malfunction in special needs children
- Developing a disaster plan for children with special needs
- Resources for emergency care providers

Chapter 8, "Including Pediatric Care Needs in Disaster Management," authored by Francine Westergaard, R.N., M.S.N., M.B.A., Mary Lacher, M.D., F.A.A.P., and Steven E. Krug, M.D., F.A.A.P., focuses on the importance of why EDs should include the needs of pediatric patients in their disaster management plans. The chapter discusses the following topics:

- Understanding the unique differences in the pediatric patient
- Addressing the needs of unaccompanied children and families
- Planning for children in a mass casualty event
- Communication
- Patient triage
- Decontamination
- Acute care capability and surge capacity
- Staff qualified to provide pediatric care

Also included, "List of Abbreviations" provides a complete list of terms and their corresponding acronyms or abbreviations used throughout the book.

How to Use the CD

Throughout *Pediatric Patient Safety in the Emergency Department,* there are checklists, forms, quick reference tables, and other tools used to enhance the care of pediatric patients in the ED. Many of these tools are included in the attached CD and may be adapted to the needs of your organization. These tools are identified throughout the book with a small CD icon.

Acknowledgements

Joint Commission Resources and the American Academy of Pediatrics gratefully acknowledge the time and insight of the following people and organizations:

- Maureen DeRosa, Director, Department of Marketing and Publications, American Academy of Pediatrics
- Linda Smessert, Manager, Clinical and Professional Publications Marketing, American Academy of Pediatrics
- Sue Tellez, Manager, Division of Hospital and Surgical Services, Department of Community and Specialty Pediatrics, American Academy of Pediatrics
- American Academy of Pediatrics Committee on Pediatric Emergency Medicine (COPEM), including:
  - Alice D. Ackerman, M.D., M.B.A., F.A.A.P.
  - Joel A. Fein, M.D., M.P.H., F.A.A.P.
  - Laura S. Fitzmaurice, M.D., F.A.A.P.
  - Susan M. Fuchs, M.D., F.A.A.P.
  - Karen S. Frush, B.S.N., M.D., F.A.A.P.
  - Louis C. Hampers, M.D., M.B.A., F.A.A.P.
  - Steven E. Krug, M.D., F.A.A.P. (Chair 2004–2008)
  - Brian R. Moore, M.D., F.A.A.P.
  - Patricia J. O'Malley, M.D., F.A.A.P.
  - Robert E. Sapien, M.D., F.A.A.P.

- Kathy N. Shaw, M.D., M.S.C.E., F.A.A.P., (Chair, 2008–2012)
- Paul E. Sirbaugh, D.O., F.A.A.P., F.A.C.E.P.
- Joseph L. Wright, M.D., M.P.H., F.A.A.P.
- Loren G. Yamamoto, M.D., M.P.H., M.B.A., F.A.A.P.

- COPEM Liaisons:
  - Kathleen Brown, M.D., American College of Emergency Physicians
  - Kim Bullock, M.D., American Academy of Family Physicians
  - Andrew Garrett, M.D., M.P.H., National Association of EMS Physicians
  - Cynthia Wright-Johnson, M.S.N., R.N., National Association of State EMS Officials
  - Dan Kavanaugh, M.S.W., Emergency Medical Services for Children Program
  - Tommy Loyacono, National Association of Emergency Medical Technicians
  - Cindy Pellegrini, AAP Department of Federal Affairs
  - Sally Snow, R.N., Emergency Nurses Association
  - David Tuggle, M.D., American College of Surgeons
  - Tina Turgel, Emergency Medical Services for Children Program
  - Tasmeen Singh Weik, DrPH, NREMTP, Emergency Medical Services for Children National Resource Center

- Chapter authors and contributors, including:
  - Coburn H. Allen, M.D., F.A.A.P.
  - Andrea T. Cruz, M.D., F.A.A.P.
  - Mary Lacher, M.D., F.A.A.P.
  - Jeannell Mansur, Pharm. D., F.A.S.H.P.
  - Richard A. Molteni, M.D., F.A.A.P.
  - Francine Westergaard, R.N., M.S.N., M.B.A.
  - Tony Woodward, M.D., M.B.A., F.A.A.P.
  - Loren G. Yamamoto, M.D., M.P.H., F.A.A.P.

- Foreword writers, including:
  - Karen S. Frush, B.S.N., M.D., F.A.A.P.
  - Edward S. Ogata, M.D., F.A.A.P.

Last but not least, we would like to extend special thanks to Steven E. Krug, M.D., F.A.A.P., for offering his expertise, talent, and tireless effort reviewing and editing the book and for authoring the preface and two chapters. We are truly grateful for his passion, patience, dedication, and tremendous contributions to the book.

References

1. McCaig L.F., Nawar E.W.: National Hospital Ambulatory Medical Care Survey: 2004 emergency department summary. *Adv Data* (372):1–29, Jul. 2006.
2. Frush K., Krug S., American Academy of Pediatrics Committee on Pediatric Emergency Medicine: Patient safety in the pediatric emergency care setting. *Pediatrics* 120:1367-1375, Dec. 2007.
3. Gaushe-Hill M., Schmitz C., Lewis R.J.: Pediatric preparedness of United States emergency departments: A 2003 survey. *Pediatrics* 120:1229–1237, Dec. 2007.
4. Institute of Medicine, Committee on Pediatric Emergency Medical Services: *Emergency medical services for children.* Washington, DC: National Academy Press, 1993.
5. Institute of Medicine, Committee on the Future of Emergency Care in the United States Health System: *Emergency care for children: growing pains.* Washington, DC: National Academy Press, 2006.
6. Hunt E.A., Hohenhaus S.M., et al.: Simulation of pediatric trauma stabilization in 35 North Carolina emergency departments: Identification of targets for performance improvement. *Pediatrics* 117:641–648, Mar. 2006.
7. Middleton K.R., Burt C.W.: Availability of pediatric services and equipment in emergency departments: United States, 2002–2003. *Adv Data* (367):1–16, Feb. 2006.
8. American Academy of Pediatrics Committee on Pediatric Emergency Medicine, American College of Emergency Physicians Pediatric Committee, Emergency Nurses Association Pediatric Committee: Guidelines for care of children in the emergency department. *Pediatrics* 124: 1233–1243, Oct. 2009.

CHAPTER 1

Hospital Leadership and Its Impact on the Care of Children in the Emergency Department

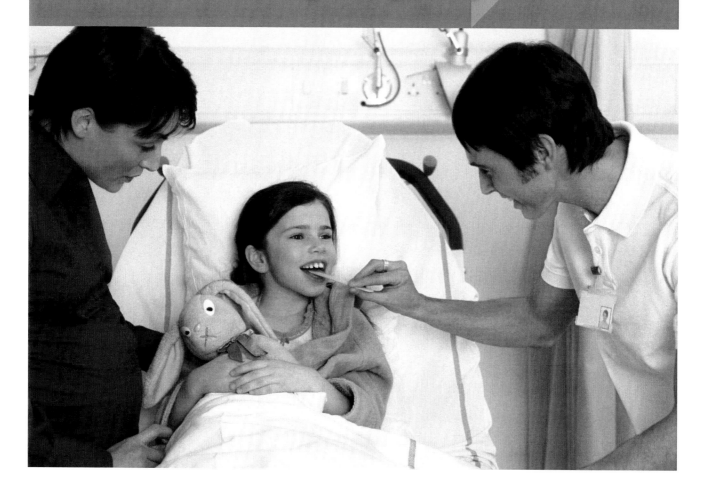

Contributing Editors: Richard A. Molteni, M.D., F.A.A.P., *intermittent consultant, Joint Commission Resources and former medical director, Seattle Children's Hospital; and* **Steven E. Krug, M.D., F.A.A.P.,** *Head of the Division of Emergency Medicine, Children's Memorial Hospital in Chicago*

It was, in short, a nightmare come true. A school bus transporting 26 children was hijacked at gunpoint. The driver and children were left to die when abandoned in a quarry. Sixteen hours later, the driver and children dug their way out and survived.[1]

Psychologists charged with debriefing the victims afterward were asked to compare their ordeal with something else that had happened to them. The children's most common response? A trip to the emergency room.[1]

This story, recounted during his pediatric emergency medicine fellowship, profoundly affected David M. Jaffe, the head of the Division of Emergency Medicine at the St. Louis Children's Hospital and the Dana Brown Professor of Pediatrics at the Washington University School of Medicine. "That day I was reminded of exactly how much work all of us had to do to address issues of pain and anxiety in pediatric emergency medicine," Jaffe says. "The emergency department can be a place of high anxiety, but through careful design and staff education we have many opportunities to reduce the risk of serious childhood and family trauma. During our brief encounter, we can have a tremendous impact on the lives of our patients and their families."[1]

For a very long time, emergency departments have well served their communities as a source of life-saving care for patients in need. The emergency department (ED) also serves as an essential component of a health care safety net, particularly for the many patients, including children, who face barriers in efforts to access care through a medical home.[2-5] More recently, for many EDs, the capacity to meet the needs of the community they serve has been challenged by rapidly expanding utilization by patients requiring both emergent and urgent care, inadequate inpatient bed capacity, and subsequent overcrowding.[6-10]

The quality of the care received by patients in the ED is greatly enhanced when it is founded on strong leadership. This often proves particularly challenging for many smaller hospitals that may not possess staff with sufficient training or experience with pediatric care. As children may represent over one quarter of all patient visits to the ED, many hospitals will be challenged in their efforts to promote patient safety and effective, timely emergency care to the children in their community.[11]

This chapter explores the role of leadership in developing a commitment to pediatric care quality and patient safety in the ED and discusses the following leadership topics: emergency medical services for children; the essential role for pediatric care leadership and advocacy in the ED; planning and budgeting for pediatric care; emphasizing training and continuing education in pediatric care; partnering with the community and building awareness; and adhering to leadership standards and guidelines for pediatric care.

Emergency Medical Services for Children (EMSC)

America's emergency medical services (EMS) systems were developed in response to the recognition of the importance of pre-hospital stabilization and hospital-based emergency care for patients with critical illness or injury in determining survival and long term outcome. The foundation for today's emergency care systems was the Emergency Medical Services Act of 1973, which promoted improvements in emergency care nationally. Despite the improvements this act brought, significant gaps remain evident, particularly for the pediatric population. These 'gaps' were the result of the inability of this emerging emergency care delivery system, with a primary orientation toward illness and injuries in adult patients, to recognize the unique anatomic, physiologic, and developmental characteristics of children, and address unique pediatric care needs. The recognition of these deficiencies ultimately prompted Federal legislation and funding for the Emergency Medical Services for Children (EMSC) program in 1985.[12,13] For more than two decades, the EMSC program has funded efforts at the state and local level to produce systematic improvements in the delivery of pediatric emergency care throughout the United States.

All emergency care professionals strive to provide children and their families with the highest quality and safest care possible. Unfortunately, significant deficiencies still exist in the pediatric care capabilities of many emergency care systems. In a 1993 report entitled, "Emergency Medical Services for Children," the Institute of Medicine (IOM) noted that many EMS systems and hospital EDs were not equally capable of caring for children and adults, and that the needs of children were frequently overlooked.[14] The IOM report noted studies demonstrating higher rates of mortality and morbidity for children versus adults treated in EDs for life-threatening events.[15,16]

A decade later, spurred by ED overcrowding and growing evidence of distress in our nation's emergency medical services, the IOM commissioned another study of the U.S. emergency care system in 2003. One segment of this three-part IOM report, published in 2006, was devoted to pediatric emergency care.[11] This report, entitled "Emergency Care for Children: Growing Pains," noted the continued presence of significant weaknesses, including insufficient pediatric emergency care training and continuing professional education for ED staff, and the absence of key pediatric equipment and medications in many EDs. The report also noted great variability in the ongoing pediatric clinical experience for both hospital and prehospital-based care providers. The report noted that only 6% of EDs had all of the equipment deemed necessary for pediatric care by the American Academy of Pediatrics and American College of Emergency Physicians.[17,18]

By the nature of their location and the community they serve, EDs vary greatly in their pediatric patient volumes, and likewise in the training, continuing education, and ongoing experience of clinical staff in the care of ill and injured children and in the available equipment to care for pediatric patients. The vast majority of children, nearly 90%, receive their emergency care in a non-children's hospital setting. Many of these visits occur in smaller, rural hospital EDs, with a quarter of pediatric visits nationwide occurring in hospital EDs that see less than 1,000 children per year, and with 50% of U.S. EDs providing care to less than 10 children a day.[19] As noted by Gausche-Hill and colleagues, EDs with larger pediatric volumes are more likely to be better prepared to care for children than EDs with smaller patient volumes.[19] Regardless of ED size, or hospital type or location, every ED must be fully prepared to provide a timely assessment and the necessary initial stabilization for an acutely ill or injured child, and likewise be able to expand its capacity in response to pediatric volume surges during winter viral epidemics, pandemics, or disasters.

The Front Door of the Hospital Organization

Improving pediatric care in an organization's ED requires well-informed, dedicated, multi-disciplinary leadership. These leaders must fully appreciate the importance and complexity of the services provided by the ED and must be able to recognize and address the ED's strengths and weaknesses. Leadership should be aware of the population served by the ED, including cultural, religious, or language needs, and be sensitive to the unique needs of at-risk populations, especially children. Leadership should be cognizant of the challenges faced by ED staff in caring for children. Through the analysis of ED pediatric care quality and patient safety outcome data at their hospital, and review of published benchmarks and guidelines for pediatric emergency care, ED leadership can then advocate for the resources, processes, and standards that will support improved readiness, care quality, and safety for children. At the very least, the care provided to children should compare well to the care provided to adults in every quality dimension and outcome.

"The ED is often the first place a family comes in contact with your facility," says Dr. Tony Woodward, Medical Director, Emergency Services; Chief, Division of Emergency Medicine at Seattle Children's Hospital. "It is their first impression of your organization. Every experience in the ED, whether it be good or bad, is a reflection of your entire organization and is invariably shared with many others in the community that you serve. In appreciating that perspective, organizational leaders should recognize that the ED doesn't work in isolation. The quality of the care and service received in the ED can easily be generalized to that expected throughout the organization."

The ED is really the front door to the hospital organization, with approximately half of the hospital's admissions entering through the ED. For both patients and community-based health care providers, a perception of the quality of care, customer service, and the overall level of excellence of your hospital is often determined indelibly at this first encounter. "Your organization's Board and CEO are ultimately responsible for the ways in which your ED is equipped, managed, and staffed," says Woodward. "It is their guidance that ensures that your ED is treated as an equal and integral unit in your system. They must empower your organization's ED leaders to take measures that uphold this principle and be proactively involved in improving the pediatric care that is provided in your ED."

Establishing a Culture of Safety and Team Approach in the ED

Leadership is essential in establishing safety as a patient care priority. Changes in the culture of the hospital, and on individual care units, cannot occur without effective leadership at all levels within the organization. For many organizations, changes have been provoked by tragic medical errors resulting in prominent adverse patient events. How leaders and organizations have chosen to respond to such events defines their understanding of the taxonomy of medical error and their view of patient safety.[20]

Adverse patient events have traditionally been attributed to the failure of an individual to perform, often to levels of expectation unattainable by any of us. James Reason has demonstrated that unplanned or unexpected patient outcomes most commonly represent a system or process defect, or a failure of communication or teamwork, rather than an individual failure.[21] Leaders must understand core safety concepts, as this will allow the transition from the "shame and blame" approach to adverse event analysis to one that focuses on the failures and resilience of systems.[22] According to the IOM, this transition to a focus on the complex microsystems that underpin our decisions rather than individual provider/patient failures is perhaps the greatest challenge facing present day health systems.[23,24] This same approach must be taken by leaders as they attempt to improve pediatric patient safety and particularly in settings with limited ongoing exposure to ill and injured children. It is only through a systematic and team-based approach to pediatric readiness that leaders can achieve improvements in care quality and patient safety for pediatric patients in the ED.[25] This approach includes leveling hierarchy and providing all staff the ability to speak up when they are uncomfortable with decisions. The ability to recognize system and process failures is very dependent on the organization's commitment to staff education, which enables them to evaluate safety events from a systems-based perspective and to apply that same rigor to the evaluation of "near misses," "close calls," or "almost" events.

Organizations that hope to sustain efforts to improve care quality and safety must support the development of a "just culture" in their hospital. A just culture requires an atmosphere of mutual trust, where staff are encouraged, and perhaps even rewarded, for providing safety-related information to their peers or managers.[20] In this same atmosphere the roles and responsibilities for leaders, managers, and front-line staff are made clear, as are expectations for professional performance and behavior. A just culture is the foundation for the evolution of a culture of safety, and may prove to be the single most effective change that an organization makes toward reducing errors and patient harm.[26]

The ED is constantly being challenged to improve its service, enhance its efficiency, and implement and sustain quality and safety improvements. To meet these critical challenges hospital leadership must rely on the skills and expertise of its ED professionals. Emergency care is a highly complex and dynamic system with many interdependent processes. This complexity makes teamwork an essential characteristic for the consistent delivery of timely, effective, and safe care. The culture and expectations for teamwork are shaped at a hospital and ED leadership level. This same culture will enable ED leadership to measure performance, and then plan for and implement change, with a goal to continually improve the services provided to patients and families. Strong local leadership, combined with the support of senior hospital management, is key in encouraging positive change.

The realities of the ED dictate variable patient care needs and volumes by time of day, day of week, and season. Leaders in the ED must similarly maintain a fluid and flexible management style and staffing patterns to adjust for these variances. Effective clinical teamwork and a culture supportive of patient safety demand bidirectional and barrier-free communication between members of the care team. This type of communication should extend beyond the staff caring for the patient in the ED to include care providers who refer to the ED and receive patients back into their practices, and healthcare professionals who accept patients for admission to the hospital. When traditional hierarchical structures are removed between physicians, nurses, and other health care professionals, and when team leaders set a tone of mutual respect and "psychological safety," communication will not be hindered by rank or limited within discipline-based "silos," alleviating conflict, reducing risk of medical error, and allowing effective change. This collaboration must exist at all levels of ED management and among frontline staff caring for patients.[25]

Although empowered by hospital leadership, ED leaders must in turn rely on their frontline team to identify quality and patient safety concerns and to assist their efforts to improve care processes and reduce the risk for medical error. The frontline team often includes ED physicians, nurses, and other clinicians (e.g., advanced practice nurses, physician assistants, respiratory care practitioners, paramedics), non-clinical ED staff (e.g., unit clerks, translators, child life), and frontline staff and administrative leadership from key support departments, such as radiology, laboratory, pharmacy, social work, and material management. Unlike other areas of the hospital, ED frontline staff and clinical managers are frequently required to be decision makers and are responsible for implementing and enforcing essential policies and procedures 24/7.

"While senior hospital leadership may plan the function and processes underpinning your emergency department, ED physician and nursing leadership must translate that plan to action and pull the frontline team together," says Matt Scanlon, M.D., patient safety program director and pediatric critical care specialist at Children's Hospital of Wisconsin–Milwaukee. "Doctors and nurses orchestrate the process at the bedside and lead the multidisciplinary team." Bedside providers are almost always a gold mine of great ideas for improving quality, safety, and efficiency. Introducing leadership walk rounds that encourage a direct dialogue between frontline staff and ED leadership can be invaluable in identifying strategies to improve quality and safety in your own ED. Celebrate reporting of errors or near miss opportunities and reward staff who begin to make this cultural transition.

A strategy to actively engage the participation of frontline staff in the identification of ED quality and patient safety issues, and efforts by leadership to reduce adverse events and improve patient outcomes and satisfaction, are Patient Safety Walk Rounds. First described by Shaw and colleagues[27] at the Children's Hospital of Philadelphia, these rounds differ from the leadership rounds model in that they are led by frontline staff. In this model, each walk-round is co-lead by an ED staff physician and nurse. The co-leaders enlist other ED frontline staff and gather live data on a variety of care quality, service excellence, and safety topics. Frontline staff are interviewed by their peers, rather than by managers, regarding their observations and concerns related to safety. Shaw and colleagues believe that this innovative approach has allowed for more open and meaningful data gathering versus the traditional leadership rounds and has inspired ED staff to actively participate in making their workplace a safer place for patients.[27]

This patient safety walk-rounds model has been adopted by ED leadership at Children's Memorial Hospital in Chicago. "We've been able to conduct these rounds about once a month, and have engaged staff from all shifts," says Steven Krug, M.D., F.A.A.P., Head of the Division of Emergency Medicine. "The walk-rounds have added significantly to the bi-directional flow of communication between ED leadership and frontline staff. The walk-rounds have helped us to identify errors, flawed patient care processes, risks for patient harm, and opportunities to improve patient and family satisfaction. They have also aided our efforts to disseminate new policies, and have promoted a substantial increase in the use of the hospital's safety event reporting system by ED staff."

Another source of wonderful advice on making our ED systems safer and the quality of care constantly higher is the patient and their family. Many families of children with chronic conditions frequently seek advice and treatment at our EDs. They look at us with different eyes and their observations can be extremely valuable in creating safer systems and processes of care.

Although all members of the health care team must be clinically competent, individual skill or expertise does not ensure competent team performance. It is only by fully understanding the effectiveness of teamwork, and modeling team behaviors, that ED managers can provide effective leadership. Teamwork training, which can include courses for staff on effective communication techniques, crew resource management (CRM), or in situ simulation, all embrace the notion that effective communication and desirable behaviors among team members can be identified, taught, and applied consistently to high-risk patient care processes.[26] Also termed "cockpit management," CRM is patterned on experiences from the aviation industry where any individual, regardless of rank or position can keep a plane on the ground until their concern is answered. In the manufacturing industry, the concept of "stop the line" similarly empowers any worker to stop an assembly line if they see a defect or the risk of a defect. In medicine, the same principle empowers any member of the ED team to halt a diagnostic procedure if they have a concern (e.g., wrong patient, wrong limb, contraindication), or to not complete an ordered treatment (e.g., not fulfill a medication order) if they perceive a patient error or immediate risk to the patient.

As suggested above, the development of an environment supportive of teamwork and open communication is a key leadership responsibility. ED leaders do this by setting expectations for professional performance and patient care processes, and then by modeling these desired behaviors. For the team to be successful, ED staff must be willing to accept input from all team members, regardless of their discipline or rank. Central to successful teamwork is the ability of members (and their commitment) to communicate effectively, in a fashion that allows the development of a shared mental model, or team cognition, a shared understanding of the clinical situation and what needs to be done.[25,28]

Supported by hospital leadership, ED leaders should establish clear expectations for teamwork behaviors. By formally establishing these teamwork expectations, each ED team member learns that he/she must not only balance the demands of their own immediate patient care responsibilities, but that they are also responsible for monitoring the activities of their fellow team members, and to maintain a situational awareness to ensure sound delivery of care. If team members engage in mutual performance monitoring, they can then provide back-up behaviors, stepping in to assist as needed, or intervene without being asked to prevent an error. If ED staff are able and willing to engage in these back-up behaviors that protect their patients, they are then able to adapt to changing needs of other team members, changes in the environment, or changes in the needs of the patient and his or her family. This adaptability is especially useful in clinical settings like the ED with high patient acuity and highly variable clinical demands.[28,29]

Effective teamwork enables organizations to set up a series of checks and balances, or "fail safe" or "default"

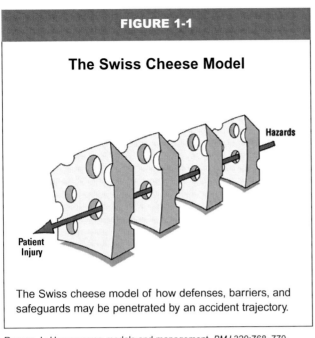

FIGURE 1-1

The Swiss Cheese Model

Hazards

Patient Injury

The Swiss cheese model of how defenses, barriers, and safeguards may be penetrated by an accident trajectory.

Reason J.: Human error: models and management. *BMJ* 320:768–770, March 2000. Printed with permission.

mechanisms that maximize safe care delivery. This redundancy in systems allows for the recognition of errors before they reach patients, or the lessening of their effect on patients. The "Swiss Cheese" model of accident causation (Figure 1-1, above), first developed by James Reason, offers an example for how such checks and balances work. The model views human systems as successive layers of "cheese" or defenses against error. The layers of cheese represent redundancy in systems, which help to prevent hazards or errors from passing through and causing harm. The holes in each layer of cheese represent inherent imperfections in each of these systems or defenses. Even with multiple layers, some hazards manage to find the right holes and bypass the defense lawyers, resulting in accidents, losses, or injuries.[21]

Periodic teamwork training is important to incorporate, reinforce, and sustain teamwork behaviors as part of the ED culture. An effective team must[30,31]:

- Educate staff on principles of safety, quality, and team behaviors

- Engage team members in planning and in decision making

- Assign clear roles and responsibilities to team members

- Offer reliable and timely data to support decision making

- Use check back processes to verify communication

- Alert members to potential biases and errors

- Listen carefully to patients, families, and each other

- Cross-monitor actions of team members

- Hold all members accountable

- Establish a just culture that encourages reporting of adverse events and "near misses"

- Debrief frequently

- Provide stress and grief support

- Maintain focused continuing education

Team data review, solution brain storming, implementation and communication strategies, and re-evaluation of effectiveness, make ED staff better able to identify specific challenges and solutions in the pediatric care they provide. Table 1-1, page 7, outlines common pediatric patient safety challenges to EDs and potential solutions to each of these challenges.

In addition to the general value of teamwork, teams can be particularly important to the quality and safety of pediatric care delivered in the community hospital ED setting. In this setting, in contrast to the pediatric-dedicated ED, teams become an effective mechanism to clarify, communicate, and leverage the pediatric expertise of all providers on the unit. Effective teams generally develop role clarity and expertise clarity, where each team member becomes well aware of the complementary roles played by others and even the strengths and weaknesses of those team members. In a setting where pediatric expertise may be limited and focused within a few individuals, strong teamwork becomes an important way to clarify: who has the expertise; the extent of the available pediatric expertise; and how these individuals' knowledge can complement other members of the team in their roles. When event debriefing indicates a gap in team knowledge, performance, or experience, it is important to turn to an internal or external expert, or a "pediatric champion," who will take accountability for professional education, team training, and process change.

The Essential Role for Pediatric Care Leadership and Advocacy in the ED

Responding to the need to enhance the day-to-day pediatric readiness of EDs, and the quality and safety of emergency care provided to children, the American Academy of Pediatrics (AAP), the American College of Emergency Physicians (ACEP), the Emergency Nurses Association (ENA), and a number of endorsing professional organizations have specified needed equipment, medications and supplies, physician and nurse qualifications, and related services that should be in place in any ED.[18,32] These published

TABLE 1-1

Challenges and Solutions in ED Pediatric Care

Challenges	Solutions
Administrative issues	
Skills of health care personnel	Orientation and training of personnel
Improper patient identification	Site identification/informed consent/time-out before procedure
Site identification	Form for children with special health care needs
Children with special health care needs	Patients rights
Advance directives	
Communication	
Emergency care transitions:	Teamwork training Emergency Team Coordination Course (ETCC) before and after:
Prehospital	Team behavior/improve behavior
Chronic care facilities	ED performance/reduce error
Sign-out/change of shift	Attitudes and opinions/improve attitudes
Information management	Work on:
	Awareness of cognitive bias
	Improving team situational awareness and communication
	Exploring systems to facilitate effective transfer of relevant information
Staff and patient/family communication	Improve staff and patient/family communication by:
	Patient and family education
	Provider and/or staff-patient communication
	Staff communication and collaboration
	Information dissemination and multidisciplinary teamwork
	Error disclosure:
	Provider-specific education
	Enhanced teamwork training
	Mechanism for disclosure of resident errors to attending physicians, patients, and families
	Disclosure of attending physician errors to patients and families
	Communication consult service
Diagnostic	
Computed tomographic reading	Teamwork training
Radiographic reading	Mechanism to report abnormal radiology readings
Abnormal laboratory results	Mechanism to report abnormal laboratory values
Documentation	
History, physical examination, procedure notes	Template charting/dictation
Legibility	
Preprocedural sedation assessment and documentation	Procedural sedation forms
Drug therapy	
Medications:	
Patient's weight	Weight in kilograms only
Dose	Near miss report/nonpunitive
Calculation error	Increase frequency of medication safety in-service sessions
10-fold error	Monitoring prescriptions to survey contents for optimum safety
Incorrect medication	Read back verbal orders
Look-alike	Bar code identification
Sound-alike	Medications administered by nurses only
Multidose formulation	
Abbreviations	
Drug allergy	
Drug interaction	
Adverse reactions	
Complications	
Pain management	Charts with preprinted pain scale
Environmental	
Physical environment	Organizational changes
Equipment use	Equipment in service
Infection control	Hand hygiene

Barata I.A., Benjamin L.S., Mace S.E., et al.: Pediatric patient safety in the prehospital/emergency department setting. *Pediatr Emerg Care* 23(6):412–418, 2007. Printed with permission.

| Sidebar 1-1 | Guidelines for the Administration of the ED for the Care of Children |

A. A Physician Coordinator for pediatric emergency medicine is appointed by the ED Medical Director.

1. **The Physician Coordinator has the following qualifications:**

   a. Meets the qualifications for credentialing by the hospital as a specialist in emergency medicine or pediatric emergency medicine. It is recognized that physicians in these specialties may not always be available in some communities; in these areas, the Physician Coordinator must meet the qualifications for credentialing by the hospital as a specialist in pediatrics or family medicine and demonstrate, through experience or continuing education, competence in the care of children in emergency settings, including resuscitation.

   b. Has special interest, knowledge, and skill in emergency medical care of children as demonstrated by training, clinical experience, or focused continuing medical education.

   c. Maintains competency in pediatric emergency care (*See* Section III of AAP, ACEP, and ENA's Guidelines for Care of Children in the Emergency Department: Quality Improvement/ Performance Improvement in the ED.).

   d. The Physician Coordinator may be a staff physician who is currently assigned other roles in the ED or may be shared through formal consultation agreements with professional resources from a hospital capable of providing definitive pediatric care.

2. **The Physician Coordinator is responsible for the following:**

   a Promote and verify adequate skill and knowledge of ED staff physicians and other ED health care providers (i.e., physician assistants and advanced practice nurses) in the emergency care and resuscitation of infants and children.

   b. Oversee ED pediatric quality improvement (QI), performance improvement (PI), patient safety, injury and illness prevention, and clinical care activities.

   c. Assist with development and periodic review of ED policies and procedures and standards for medications, equipment, and supplies to assure adequate resources for children of all ages.

   d. Serve as liaison/coordinator to appropriate in-hospital and out-of-hospital pediatric care committees in the community (if they exist).

   e. Serve as liaison/coordinator to a definitive care hospital (such as a regional pediatric referral hospital and trauma center), EMS agencies, primary care providers, health insurers, and any other medical resources needed to integrate services for the continuum of care of the pediatric patient.

   f. Facilitate pediatric emergency education for ED health care providers and out-of-hospital providers affiliated with the ED.

   g. Ensure that competency evaluations completed by the staff are pertinent to children of all ages.

   h. Ensure pediatric needs are addressed in hospital disaster/emergency preparedness plans.

   i. Collaborate with the nursing coordinator to ensure adequate staffing, medications, equipment, supplies, and other resources for children in the ED.

B. A Nursing Coordinator for pediatric emergency care is appointed by the ED Nursing Director.

1. **The Nursing Coordinator has the following qualifications:**

   a. Registered nurse (RN) possessing special interest, knowledge, and skill in the emergency medical care of children as demonstrated by training, clinical experience, or focused continuing nursing education.

   b. Maintains competency in pediatric emergency care.

   c. Credentialed and has competency verification per the hospital policies and guidelines to provide care to children of all ages.

   d. The Nursing Coordinator may be a staff nurse who is currently assigned other roles in the ED, such as Clinical Nurse Specialist, or may be shared through formal consultation agreements with professional resources from a hospital capable of providing definitive pediatric care.

(Continued on next page)

Guidelines for the Administration of the ED for the Care of Children (continued)

2. **The Nursing Coordinator is responsible for the following:**

   a. Facilitate ED pediatric QI/PI activities. (*See* Section III of AAP, ACEP, and ENA's Guidelines for Care of Children in the Emergency Department: Quality Improvement/Performance Improvement in the ED.)

   b. Serve as liaison to appropriate in-hospital and out-of-hospital pediatric care committees.

   c. Serve as liaison to inpatient nursing as well as to a definitive care hospital, a regional pediatric referral hospital and trauma center, EMS agencies, primary care providers, health insurers, and any other medical resources needed to integrate services for the continuum of care of the pediatric patient.

   d. Facilitate, along with hospital-based educational activities, ED nursing continuing education in pediatrics and ensure that pediatric-specific elements are included in orientation for new staff members.

   e. Ensure initial and annual competency evaluations completed by the nursing staff are pertinent to children of all ages.

   f. Promote pediatric disaster preparedness for the ED and participate in hospital disaster preparedness activities.

   g. Promote patient and family education in illness and injury prevention.

   h. Provide assistance and support for pediatric education of out-of-hospital providers affiliated with the ED.

   i. Work with clinical leadership to ensure the availability of pediatric equipment, medications, staffing, and other resources through the development and periodic review of ED standards, policies, and procedures.

   j. Collaborate with the physician coordinator to ensure that the ED is prepared to care for children of all ages, including children with special health care needs.

American Academy of Pediatrics Committee on Pediatric Emergency Medicine, American College of Emergency Physicians Pediatric Committee, Emergency Nurses Association Pediatric Committee: Guidelines for care of children in the emergency department. *Pediatrics* 124: 1233–1243, Oct. 2009. Printed with permission.

recommendations offer useful guidelines for the components necessary for optimal emergency care and stress the importance that these elements relate to one another to form a more comprehensive and effective pediatric care delivery system.

Championed by the federal Emergency Medical Services for Children (EMSC) program,[33] and consistent with Recommendation 3.1 in the 2006 IOM report,[11] these guidelines for pediatric emergency preparedness have formed the foundation of a categorization system for EDs based on pediatric service capabilities. A handful of model hospital designation programs, both voluntary and legislated, for pediatric emergency care have been implemented by individual state EMSC programs.[33-35] Although there is not yet data demonstrating improved patient outcomes, pediatric emergency experts believe that EDs meeting these standards, also known as "EDAPs" (Emergency Departments Approved for Pediatrics), are better prepared and offer optimal patient outcomes.

From a pediatric leadership and advocacy standpoint, these guidelines recommend that hospital organizations consider an ED administrative structure to include both a Physician Coordinator and a Nursing Coordinator for pediatric care. Sidebar 1-1 outlines the roles and qualifications of these positions.[32]

As described in the AAP/ACEP/ENA guidelines, the pediatric care expert or champion role would be filled by the Physician and Nursing Coordinators. The ED leadership team in a non-children's hospital setting can benefit significantly from identifying pediatric expertise to assist their efforts to promote care quality and patient safety for children. If not readily available within ED leadership or staff, this expertise may be found in other hospital departments (e.g., inpatient pediatrics, neonatology, family medicine), in the community (e.g., office-based pediatrician or family physician), or perhaps at a local or regional pediatric specialty care center. The ED leadership team may likewise be further strengthened by assigning a qualified

Sidebar 1-2	Purpose and Suggested Functions of a LILY Team

Purpose

A LILY Team evaluates and improves the capability and plans for treating children in the ED and includes evidence-based approaches to reduce errors in emergency and trauma care for children. A LILY Team can play a pivotal role in developing and leading emergency management processes for pediatric patients.

Team Membership

A LILY Team may include pediatricians, family physicians, emergency medicine physicians, ED nurses, pediatric nurses (when possible), a pharmacist, an infection control practitioner, the ED administrator, a parent from the community, and others.

Suggested Team Functions

Clinical Care

- Develop triage protocols that are pediatric age- and symptom- or diagnosis-specific, including a process for identifying children with special health care needs.
- Review and recommend approval and implementation of pediatric-specific evidence-based treatment protocols.
- Evaluate variances in performance and adherence to clinical pathways.
- Develop, implement, monitor compliance with, and update policies and procedures related to the care of pediatric patients in the ED.
- Establish principles of patient- and family-centered care and monitor adherence.
- Respond to patient/family/provider staff concerns regarding quality, safety, or service.

Emergency Department Utilization and Disaster Planning

- Develop a strategy for responding to a surge of pediatric patients during a disaster or pandemic in the community; participate in the development of hospital and community disaster plans to assure that the needs of children are incorporated into all-hazard planning and in all plan aspects (e.g., surveillance, triage, decontamination, treatment, sheltering), including surge capacity plans sufficient to meet the needs of ill and injured children in excess of the usual number of children treated by the ED.

- Participate in hospital and community activities focused on ameliorating overcrowding, work to assure optimal patient flow inside and outside of the ED to assure that pediatric care is not compromised.

Equipment, Supplies, and Space

- Assure that the ED space is family-friendly and a physically safe environment to care for children of all ages.
- Conduct a needs assessment to develop equipment and supply checklists that conform to the ED's approach to patient age- and size-specific pediatric care.
- Participate in the development of the ED's budget to assure required resources (staff, equipment, and supplies) are available to provide safe care, consistent with published guidelines (AAP/ACEP/ENA).
- Ensure/conduct routine scheduled checks of pediatric equipment, medications, and supplies, the ED environment, to ensure they are pediatric-appropriate and well-maintained.
- Assure that equipment is well-organized and easily accessed for treating pediatric patients.
- Review equipment and medications on the code carts.
- Establish a pediatric resuscitation/code cart. If combined adult/pediatric code carts are utilized be certain that medication doses and storage practices minimize the risk for the use of adult drugs or concentrations in small children.
- Hold mock pediatric codes on a scheduled basis.
- Conduct immediate debriefings and review of all codes, including mock codes.
- Designate a safe treatment area where pediatric care will take place.
- Establish a family and child friendly environment (furnishings, fixtures, availability of toys, and play activities).

Patient/Family Education and Community Outreach

- Recruit and/or contribute articles to internal and external newsletters related to the safe care of children and illness and injury prevention.
- Periodically conduct surveys and open forums with families and community physicians to assess their satisfaction with the ED's care of children.

(Continued on next page)

Sidebar 1-2	**Purpose and Suggested Functions of a LILY Team** (continued)

- Ensure that patient satisfaction surveys address the ED's care of pediatric patients and utilize results to drive change as indicated.

Quality Measurement and Performance Improvement

- Participate in developing the ED's mission, vision, and philosophy of care statements to include the care of children.

- Recommend performance improvement projects based on data observed and measured pediatric care in the ED and driven by pediatric-specific performance measures.

- Provide leadership and become a champion in quality measurement and improvement activities to enhance care of pediatric patients in the ED.

- Collaborate with hospital accreditation staff to ensure external standards and regulations are met.

- Work closely with the hospital infection control coordinator to minimize the risk of transmission of infection to and from patients and families.

Staff Knowledge, Education, and Competency

- Outline education and training needs for ED staff that care for pediatric patients.

- Monitor competency evaluations of ED staff that care for pediatric patients.

- Respond to performance measurement data that indicates the need for new policies, staff education, or re-training of ED staff that care for pediatric patients.

- Conduct periodic education programs to keep ED staff updated on current, evidence-based emergency care for pediatric patients of all ages.

Pediatric Patient Safety Consulting Service, Joint Commission Resources © 2008.

ED team member (a nurse and/or physician) the role of pediatric champion. This designation empowers a team member to advocate for pediatric quality and safety—in effect being the voice for pediatrics. The general importance of quality champions is well established in the literature. In a setting where pediatric quality needs may not be well understood or consistently attended to, a champion for pediatric care becomes even more important. The dynamic link between the ongoing review of pediatric patient care, the analysis of medical errors and adverse events, and continuing education and process improvement is essential even for EDs located in pediatric specialty hospitals.

The designation of a pediatric champion is also a leadership issue in two respects. First, the champion becomes a local leader for all pediatric emergency care provided in the institution, especially when more formal leaders, such as a department head, may not be on the unit. It is also a leadership issue for managers and senior leaders who can support pediatric quality and safety by ensuring that (1) there is a designated pediatric champion, (2) the recognized champion is supported by peers and managers, and (3) the champion has the resources and skills needed to do the job. In a 2003 survey examining the pediatric readiness of U.S. EDs, the presence of a pediatric coordinator was associated with improved pediatric readiness and care quality, regardless of ED size or location.[19] It merits noting that the AAP/ACEP/ENA guidelines are intended to apply to hospital-based EDs with 24/7 physician staffing. Hospitals without 24/7 physician staffing in their ED (so called "standby hospitals"), or free-standing EDs, may be unable to institute the full scope of these guidelines. They are still encouraged to comply with as many of these recommendations as is reasonable and possible. Perhaps the best place to start would be by identifying a pediatric care champion.

Forming a LILY Team

The physician and nursing coordinators for pediatrics should lead the formation of a Lifesaving Interventions for Little Youth (LILY) team. A LILY team evaluates and improves the capability and plans for treating children in the ED and includes evidence-based approaches to reduce errors in emergency and trauma care for children.[36] The LILY team would include the following members:

TABLE 1-2

Guidelines for Equipment and Supplies for Use with Pediatric Patients in the ED

General Equipment

- Patient warming device
- IV blood/fluid warmer
- Restraint device
- Weight scale, in kilograms only (no pounds), for infants and children
- Tool or chart that incorporates both weight (in kilograms) and length to assist physicians and nurses in determining equipment size and correct drug dosing (by weight and total volume), such as a length-based resuscitation tape
- Pain scale assessment tools appropriate for age

Monitoring Equipment

- Blood pressure cuffs (neonatal, infant, child, adult-arm, and thigh)
- Doppler ultrasonography
- ECG monitor/defibrillator with pediatric and adult dose capabilities including pediatric-sized pads/paddles
- Hypothermia thermometer
- Pulse oximeter with pediatric and adult probes
- Continuous end-tidal CO_2 monitoring device[a]

Respiratory Equipment and Supplies

- Endotracheal tubes:
  - (uncuffed: 2.5, 3.0 mm)
  - (cuffed or uncuffed: 3.5, 4.0, 4.5, 5.0, 5.5 mm)
  - (cuffed: 6.0, 6.5, 7.0, 7.5, 8.0 mm)
- Feeding tubes (5F, 8F)

- Laryngoscope blades (curved: 2,3; straight: 0, 1, 2, 3)
- Laryngoscope handle
- Magill forceps (pediatric and adult)
- Nasopharyngeal airways (infant, child, and adult)
- Oropharyngeal airways (sizes 0–5)
- Stylettes for endotracheal tubes (pediatric and adult)
- Suction catheters (infant, child, and adult)
- Tracheostomy tubes (tube sizes 0–6)
- Yankauer suction tip
- Bag-mask device (manual resuscitator); self-inflating (infant size: 450 mL; adult size: 1000 mL)
- Clear oxygen masks (standard and non-rebreathing) for an infant, child, and adult
- Masks to fit bag-mask device adaptor (neonatal, infant, child, and adult sizes)
- Nasal cannulae (infant, child, and adult)
- Nasogastric tubes: infant (8F), child (10F), and adult (14F–18F)
- Laryngeal mask airway[b] (sizes 1, 1.5, 2, 2.5, 3, 4, and 5)

Vascular Access Supplies and Equipment

- Arm boards (infant, child, and adult sizes)
- Catheter over the needle (14–24 gauge)
- Intraosseous needles or device (pediatric and adult sizes)

- IV administration sets with calibrated chambers and extension tubing and/or infusion devices with ability to regulate rate and volume of infusate
- Umbilical vein catheters (3.5F and 5.0F)[c]
- Central venous catheters (4.0F–7.0F)
- IV solutions to include: NS; D5 0.45% NS; and D10W

Fracture Management Devices

- Extremity splints, including femur splints (pediatric and adult sizes)
- Spine stabilization method/devices appropriate for children of all ages[d]

Specialized Pediatric Trays or Kits

- Lumbar puncture tray including infant (22 gauge), pediatric (22 gauge), and adult (18–21 gauge) lumbar puncture needles
- Supplies/kit for patients with difficult airway conditions (to include but not limited to supraglottic airways of all sizes, such as the laryngeal mask airway, needle cricothyrotomy supplies, or surgical cricothyrotomy kit)
- Tube thoracostomy tray
- Chest tubes to include infant, child, and adult sizes (infant: 8F–12F; child: 14F–22F; adult: 24F–40F)
- Newborn delivery kit (including equipment for initial resuscitation of a newborn infant: umbilical clamp, scissors, bulb syringe, and towel)
- Urinary catheterization kits and urinary (indwelling) catheters (6F–22F)

IV indicates intravenous; ECG, electrocardiography; CO_2, carbon dioxide; F, French; NS, normal saline; D5 0.45% NS, 5% dextrose in 45% normal saline; D10W, 10% dextrose in water.

a End-tidal CO_2 monitoring is considered the optimal method of assessing for and monitoring of endotracheal tube placement in the trachea; however, for low-volume hospitals, adult and pediatric CO_2 colorimetric detector devices could be substituted. Clinical assessment alone is not appropriate.

b Laryngeal mask airways could be shared with anesthesia but must be immediately accessible to the ED.

c Feeding tubes (size 5F) may be utilized as umbilical venous catheters but are not ideal. A method to secure the umbilical catheter, such as an umbilical tie, should also be available.

d A spinal stabilization device should be a device that can also stabilize the neck of an infant, child, or adolescent in a neutral position.

American Academy of Pediatrics Committee on Pediatric Emergency Medicine, American College of Emergency Physicians Pediatric Committee, Emergency Nurses Association Pediatric Committee: Guidelines for care of children in the emergency department. *Pediatrics* 124:1233–1243, Oct. 2009. Printed with permission.

- Pediatricians and/or family physicians
- Emergency medicine physicians
- Emergency department nurses
- Pediatric nurses (when possible)
- Pharmacist(s)
- Infection control practitioner(s)
- ED administrator(s)
- Parent(s) from the community
- Former pediatric patients as advocates

The purpose and suggested functions of a LILY Team are further discussed in Sidebar 1-2 on page 10.

Planning and Budgeting for Pediatric Care

Although an effective administrative structure establishes clinical cohesion and communication between the ED and support departments such as pharmacy, radiology or laboratory, it is essential that these departments are capable of safely meeting the needs of children being cared for in the ED. The radiology department can safely and effectively provide needed imaging studies for children only if it has the proper equipment, imaging, and safety protocols, and skilled personnel. The clinical laboratory can perform laboratory tests for children of all ages if it has the equipment and skilled personnel necessary to do so. The pharmacy requires adequate staffing to be able to review all medications used in the ED and prepare weight-based pediatric formulations that may be unfamiliar to ED staff or those that present particular risk to small patients. Organizations must consider and budget for the special equipment and staff training and education necessary to treat pediatric patients across departments.

Meeting the special needs of pediatric patients in the ED in many hospitals means purchasing and maintaining expensive and infrequently used equipment and supplies that are essential to safely care for children of all ages, including sizes appropriate for premature infants through adolescents. Additionally, staff need to know what equipment to use and then receive training on when and how to use it. Each organization should also develop a method for storage that provides an easily visible and accessible site for infrequently used medications and pediatric-sized equipment, as well as a policy for restocking and replacing expired medications and equipment. EDs should provide tools (e.g., length-based tape dosing guide, manuals, or web-based resources containing pre-calculated drug doses and equipment sizes for specific patient weights)

to assist ED staff in the selection of the appropriate doses of medications and sizes of equipment for children of all ages. Table 1-2, page 12, lists equipment and supplies recommended by the AAP, ACEP, and ENA for use in pediatric patients in the ED.[32] Mock codes and other similar practice sessions will assure that staff know where this equipment is located, what sizes are appropriate for children of various ages, and which medications and doses are indicated for pediatric emergencies.

Organizations should routinely conduct needs assessments and develop equipment and supply checklists that conform to the ED's approach to patient care and the population of children served. These assessments should examine areas of vulnerability and include patient tracer methodology to evaluate the efficiency of processes and procedures. Analysis of data from safety event reporting systems may assist in the identification of vulnerabilities, though many near misses and even adverse patient events may go unreported. Increasing the reporting of these events is the responsibility of ED leaders and pediatric champions as they move their department's safety culture from "blame and shame" to "opportunity to improve." It is essential that ED leaders recognize gaps in care before they are faced with a serious or sentinel event. Although most EDs primarily care for adults, even those that do not see a high volume of children should make the care of pediatric patients a central focus for quality improvement. The lower the volume of pediatric patients served and the less familiar the ED staff are with pediatric equipment, the more critical is this need.

Emphasizing Training and Continuing Education in Pediatric Care

In budgeting for an ED that is prepared to treat children, organizations must also consider the need for additional training of clinical staff in the evaluation and management of pediatric patients. It is essential that physicians and nurses staffing the ED have the necessary skill, knowledge, and training to provide emergency assessment and treatment for children of all ages who may be brought to the ED, consistent with the services provided by the hospital. Physician and nursing coordinators for pediatric care should prove useful as advocates, and perhaps even as providers, for targeted continuing professional education, and in the assessment of staff competencies in pediatric care. Developing a relationship that supports consultation and continuing education from a regional hospital that provides large volume and high intensity pediatric care or a regional children's hospital will make this responsibility much easier to accomplish.

It is ultimately the responsibility of ED leadership to assure that their staff is well trained and maintains competency in the treatment of all patients that present to their ED. Organizations should develop a clearly defined mechanism to monitor professional education and clinical competency. Leaders should also ensure that competency evaluations completed by the staff are specific to the following age groups:

- Neonates
- Infants
- Toddlers
- Children
- Adolescents
- Adults with congenital conditions and defects

Most general and community hospital ED staff are eager for additional pediatric educational opportunities, but, is there room in the ED budget to provide for staff education in pediatric patient assessment or for infrequently used pediatric-sized equipment and supplies? Is the ED properly staffed to effectively manage the volume of pediatric patients? Does the organization have available or budget for a pediatric consultant or pediatric medical or surgical subspecialists? If there are gaps in the availability of pediatric consultants, does the hospital have a plan for the safe and timely transfer of children to an appropriate facility where such services are available? Does the ED have strategies in place to respond to a surge of pediatric patients due to a pandemic or disaster in their community? It is incumbent upon ED leaders to assess these issues and exert their influence in the planning and budgeting processes.

This may be a difficult proposition when you consider changes in the status of healthcare delivery systems over the past decade. Most EDs have experienced a significant increase in patient volume as a result of regional population growth, decreased access to primary and specialty care physicians, and insufficient inpatient beds. Increasing numbers of uninsured or underinsured patients, including immigrants and homeless populations that are forced to use the ED as their primary source of care, adds a further burden. Even more perplexing is the observation from a 2006 IOM report that the significant increase in ED visits between 1993 and 2003 had been matched by a significant reduction in the number of EDs nationwide.[9] The ED overcrowding crisis has been likened to the canary in the coal mine, a harbinger of distress in the much larger U.S. healthcare delivery system.[5]

Addressing Emergency Department Overcrowding

ED overcrowding is one of the greatest challenges that hospitals confront today. Prior to the release of the 2006 IOM report, overcrowding was believed to primarily affect larger urban medical centers.[4-7] The IOM report demonstrated that overcrowding was much more prevalent, with more than 90% of all hospitals reporting this to be a problem, and 40% reporting it as a daily concern.[9] Overcrowding forces many EDs to divert incoming ambulances. The IOM noted that 70% of urban hospitals reported going on diversion and estimated that there were nearly 500,000 ambulance diversions in 2003, or approximately one every minute.[9] Ambulance diversion is the ultimate access barrier for ill or injured patients as it results in significantly longer transit times to the ED. In addition to access concerns, ED overcrowding is also associated with a lower quality of care and increased medical error and, in academic settings, with lower teaching quality.[5,10] Table 1-3 lists a variety of factors that contribute to ED overcrowding.

In terms of regulatory and policy issues, an analysis by the IOM in 2000 put Medicaid reimbursement policies at the top of the list of causes in the development of critical ED overcrowding.[37] This issue was highlighted by Hostetler and colleagues in a 2007 review article on ED overcrowding.[10] The authors observe that hospital restructuring in recent years has resulted in fewer inpatient beds, increased ambulatory services, and closures of hospitals or EDs. They also note that despite rising utilization of the ED, many health care organizations have not increased the amount of ED space, personnel, or equipment to keep pace with growth and may prefer to allocate limited hospital resources to other more lucrative clinical units. "Rather than implementing methods to reduce overcrowding, many [hospital administrators] intentionally choose to limit the accessibility for admissions through the ED," the authors state.[10] Part of the issue here may be a historical bias regarding patients admitted through the ED, who may be of a lower socioeconomic class and under-insured in comparison with patients directly admitted by their primary care provider. In addition, many elective surgical admissions provide a greater financial contribution (revenue per case) than most patients admitted through the ED.[5,10]

Nationwide, the numbers of EDs and hospital beds have decreased through the downsizing of hospitals, ED closures, and merging of health care institutions. The IOM noted a reduction of nearly 200,000 inpatient beds between 1993 and 2003.[9] Risk management studies have indicated that overcrowding poses a considerable risk for medical errors and adverse patient events. Children may be particularly exposed to this increased error risk because of their unique diseases and physiologic characteristics, developmental immaturity and limited communication skills, size variability and the need for age- and weight-based medication dosing, and the relative lack of pediatric experience for many emergency care providers.[10,25,32] If children are competing for the limited availability of ED care, then their access to care may be hampered even further. This may be especially problematic for the medically complex and children with special health care needs, and particularly as overcrowding also impacts tertiary pediatric referral centers.[5]

Children invariably require increased time and resources while in the ED for diagnostic studies such as laboratory testing, radiological imaging, consultations, and therapeutic interventions or procedures. Medication preparation and administration for children can also be time consuming and is a common source of error and adverse events, particularly in general ED settings. With rising numbers of children with special needs, the overall complexity of patients presenting to EDs has also increased. The increasing percentage of uninsured or underinsured ED patients, combined with poor reimbursement for mandated emergency services, has made providing the increasing numbers and complexity of those services proportionately more costly to both hospitals and community providers.[38]

In May 2003, the Joint Commission issued a proposed standard requiring a series of patient flow improvements in ED patient management to reduce the odds of harmful or fatal treatment delays occurring as a result of ED overcrowding. The proposal grew out of a national symposium on ED overcrowding and a summary of 50 deaths. The standard, which took effect in January 2005, expands responsibility for overcrowding beyond the ED to all departments within the hospital. Accountability now resides throughout the hospital in all departments and care units in which patients are held, transferred, and discharged at any point during a hospital stay. It is believed that this standard will be helpful by increasing hospitals' awareness of this problem, akin to disaster preparedness, and thereby aid in the sharing and assuming of responsibility and accountability throughout an entire organization.

One of the first priorities to improve overcrowding in the ED is optimizing use of available resources. Although a certain percentage of acutely ill or injured pediatric patients

---

TABLE 1-3

Emergency Department Overcrowding: Contributing Factors

- Overall increase in patient volume
- Increased ED utilization rates
- Increased consumer demand and expectations (such as procedural sedation)
- Increased acuity of patients presenting to the ED
- Increased complexity of ED patients (such as children with special health care needs)
- Avoidance of inpatient hospital admission by "intensive therapy" in the ED
- Lack of beds for patients requiring admission
- Lack of physical space within the ED
- Delays in service provided by radiology, laboratory, and ancillary services
- Shortage of nursing staff
- Shortage of on-call specialty and subspecialty consultant services or lack of availability (internal or external)
- Shortage of emergency medicine/pediatric emergency medicine staff
- Shortage of house staff who rotate through teaching hospital EDs related to the 80-hour work week
- Shortage of administrative, clerical, or other support staff or resources
- Increased medical record documentation requirements
- Problems with language and cultural barriers
- Lack of access to primary care/specialty care/managed care providers
- Difficulty in arranging follow-up care

Adapted from Hostetler M.A., Mace S.E., Brown K., et al.: Emergency department overcrowding and children, *Pediatr Emerg Care* 23(7):507–515, 2007.

---

are of high acuity, the majority may be of lower acuity and may arrive during predictable peak periods; most notably during evening and weekend hours. Knowing these characteristics and optimizing staffing patterns to reflect patient acuity and arrival patterns can greatly improve resource utilization. The use of midlevel providers in urgent care settings during peak hours, for example, has been found to be particularly effective at alleviating the stress caused by higher-volume, lower-acuity patients.[10]

TABLE 1-4

Emergency Department Overcrowding: Approaches to Amelioration

1. **Optimize systems to increase efficiency**
   a. Emergency department
      i. Triage protocols (pediatric-specific)
      ii. Clinical treatment guidelines (pediatric-specific)
   b. Ancillary support services
      i. Service recovery and accountability
   c. Administration/institution
      i. Early alert bed warning system
      ii. Facilitate discharge and admission process
   d. Community
      i. Clinic referrals, follow-up, and communication

2. **Optimize supply and demand within the ED**
   a. Nursing phone triage
   b. Urgent care
   c. Observation units
   d. Mid-level providers

3. **Optimize supply and demand outside the ED**
   a. Primary/specialty care referral clinics
   b. Return visits

4. **Optimize ED reimbursement**
   a. Billing and coding
   b. Coordination with hospital administration

5. **Advocacy—proactively work toward removing barriers**
   a. Improved reimbursement (policy/legislative)
   b. Improved work environment
   c. Staffing shortages
   d. Space/physical plant restrictions
   e. Administrative and political legitimacy
   f. Improved infrastructure for electronic data monitoring

Adapted from Hostetler M.A., Mace S., Brown K., et al.: Emergency department overcrowding and children, *Pediatr Emerg Care* 23(7): 507–515, 2007.

Although the issue of overcrowding in the ED is examined further in the pages ahead, Table 1-4 (above) lists other approaches for leaders to consider in dealing with the problem.[10]

Emergency department managers should also consider the optimal use of resource intensive nursing or physician patient call-backs, or brief return visits to the ED versus referral to urgent care and other outpatient sites for follow-up. It is well worth the time and energy to proactively develop ambulatory follow-up and referral relationships with both hospital and community-based primary and subspecialty care providers. This planning should encompass an awareness of provider availability and hours of service, addressing the access and service needs of the patient, community, and the hospital system.

Partnering with the Community and Building Awareness

In an effort to offset unnecessary costs associated with ED visits of low intensity and to improve the quality of pediatric care, ED leaders should consider the other ways in which they can collaborate with the community they serve. This involves thinking more broadly about the care that they provide and the potential of providing patients and families with educational interventions designed to improve disease management or prevent recurrence of illness or injury.

Through the use of newsletters or e-newsletters, community bulletin boards, community websites, and other unique forums, EDs can raise awareness about specific issues and promote the important message that children and parents should play an active role in their own health care. Community outreach programs such as health fairs are a common method of alerting families about safety issues with which ED personnel are all too familiar. For example, using child safety seats for infants and booster seats for preschoolers significantly reduces the risk for injury or death when in motor vehicle accidents.[39,40] Likewise, when bicycle helmets are used, they may reduce the risk of head injuries by as much as 85%.[41] Additionally, community outreach programs may involve education around safe gun storage and the hazards, water safety, and warning signs associated with childhood substance abuse. Offering educational interventions on issues such as these by working with community-based groups is preventative rather than reactive and can help avert future injuries. Families and patients should also be encouraged to use reliable source web-based medical advice, especially concerning influenza and other common illnesses during winter viral season and injuries during the summer months. This same strategy may serve to reduce fear and could promote more appropriate utilization of the ED by the community during peak seasons or pandemics.

These approaches can also enhance the visibility of an organization with the community that it serves, perhaps leading to further educational opportunities through the media and legislative advocacy.[42] Organizations should also develop a plan for outreach from ED staff to referring physicians in order to build stronger relationships and future referrals.

Providing Educational Interventions

In addition to ED leaders reaching outside of the organization and into the community, some have suggested that an ED visit in itself is a teachable moment for the patient and their family and in some cases the primary care provider (PCP). In most EDs, injuries account for as much as one-third of pediatric patient visits. Emergency physicians care for injuries of all severities and understand injuries as a disease process, making them ideally suited to discuss prevention, and making an ED visit an opportune time to introduce or even reemphasize injury prevention and immunization education.[42]

There are those who have expressed concern that an increase in personnel effort and time that an educational intervention might necessitate is not justifiable in an era of long wait times and overcrowded EDs. They may argue that prevention is the role of the child's medical home but, again, more and more families are turning to the ED for aspects of their primary care. Through educational intervention programs, ED physicians can enhance rather than replace the role of the medical home provider in areas of prevention, education, and counseling.

From a budgetary standpoint, injury prevention programs have demonstrated net cost savings by reducing the health care costs of averted injuries. In one study of a smoke detector giveaway program in Oklahoma City, the medical net savings were estimated at $1 million.[43] Another study demonstrated how a motorcycle helmet law nationwide could save approximately $61 million annually.[44] Prevention programs have also proven to be cost effective in lower socioeconomic groups such as Native Americans, demonstrating their value in populations with limited resources similar to those seen in many urban EDs.[42]

Ideally, the time spent by ED staff participating in ED-based intervention programs must be considered an "investment" in the health and well-being of the community served, one that over time may lead to lower utilization rates and improved ED efficiency. These activities would then be explicitly valued as an important part of a physician's or nurse's job, not something done in one's free time. Similarly, the cost savings realized from injuries averted could be reinvested by payers into the health care system in the form of reimbursement for physician time spent in counseling or other prevention activities, as well as in support of the materials that are often needed by specific prevention programs.[42]

Adhering to Leadership Standards and Guidelines for Pediatric Care

The Joint Commission has developed standards that focus on leadership and the leadership structure. These standards describe the overall responsibility of the governing body working consistently and openly with senior management and the medical staff to enhance the safety and quality of care, treatment, and services provided by all of these individuals. Likewise, the AAP, ACEP, ENA, and the EMSC program have developed standards dedicated to emergency care concerning pediatric patients. The goal of all of these standards is to ensure that quality care is delivered in the ED, among other health care settings. For more information about these standards, please use the following online resources:

- Joint Commission—www.jointcommission.org
- American Academy of Pediatrics—www.aap.org
- American College of Emergency Physicians— www.acep.org
- Emergency Nurses Association—www.ena.org
- Emergency Medical Services for Children National Resource Center—http://bolivia.hrsa.gov/emsc/

In thinking more broadly, and from a patient perspective, organizational leaders along with ED managers and frontline leaders need to continually assess the quality and scope of care that the ED provides. For example, should influenza or other immunizations be administered in the ED? Do ED leadership and members of the multi-disciplinary team agree with the extent of high volume or high-risk treatment processes? Do they recognize any gaps in care? Leadership is key in defining the issues, discovering solutions, and implementing changes that enhance the safety and quality of pediatric care.

References

1. Leydig K.: An incredible impact: David M. Jaffe advances pediatric emergency medicine across the world. *The Record* (Washington University in St. Louis), 29(5), Sep. 10, 2004. Available at: http://record.wustl.edu/news/page/normal/3763.html (accessed Dec. 5, 2008).

2. Richardson L.D., Hwang U.: America's health care safety net: intact or unraveling? *Acad Emerg Med* 8:1056–1063, 2001.

3. Adams J.G., Biros M.H.: The endangered safety net: establishing a measure of control. *Acad Emerg Med* 8:1013–1015, 2001.

4. Richardson L.D., Asplin B.R., Lowe R.A.: Emergency department crowding as a health policy issue. *Ann Emerg Med* 40:388–393, 2002.

5. Krug S.E., American Academy of Pediatrics Committee on Pediatric Emergency Medicine: Overcrowding crisis in our nation's emergency departments. Is our safety net unraveling? *Pediatrics* 114:878–888, 2004.

6. Derlet R.W., Richards J.R., Kravitz R.L.: Frequent overcrowding in U.S. emergency departments. *Acad Emerg Med* 8:151–155, 2001.

7. Derlet R.W., Richards J.R.: Overcrowding in the nation's emergency departments: complex causes and disturbing effects. *Ann Emerg Med* 35:63–68, 2000.

8. Schafermeyer R.W., Asplin B.R.: Hospital and emergency department overcrowding in the United States. Emerg Med 13:22–27, 2003.

9. Institute of Medicine, Committee on the Future of Emergency Care in the United States Health System: *Hospital-based emergency care: at the breaking point.* Washington, D.C.: National Academy Press, 2006.

10. Hostetler M.A., Mace S.E., Brown K., et al.: Emergency department overcrowding and children. *Pediatr Emerg Care* 23(7):507–515, 2007.

11. Institute of Medicine, Committee on the Future of Emergency Care in the United States Health System: *Emergency care for children: growing pains.* Washington, D.C.: National Academy Press, 2006.

12. Krug S., Kuppermann N.: Twenty years of emergency medical services for children: a cause for celebration and a call for action. *Pediatrics* 115(4):1089–1091, 2005.

13. Ball J.W., Liao E., Kavanaugh D., Turgel C.: The emergency medical services for children program: accomplishments and contributions. *Clin Pediatr Emerg Med* 7:6–14, 2006.

14. Institute of Medicine, Committee on Pediatric Emergency Medical Services: *Emergency medical services for children.* Washington, D.C.: National Academy Press, 1993.

15. Barden R., Kinscherff R., George W. III, et al.: Emergency care and injury/illness prevention systems for children. *Harvard Journal on Legislation* 30(2):467–479, 1993.

16. Seidel J.S., Henderson D.P., Yoshiyama K., et al.: Emergency medical services and the pediatric patient: are the needs being met? *Pediatrics* 73:769–772, 1984.

17. Middleton K.R., Burt C.W.: *Availability of pediatric services and equipment in emergency departments: United States, 2002–2003. Advance data from vital and health statistics;* no. 367. Hyattsville, MD: National Center for Health Statistics, 2006.

18. American Academy of Pediatrics Committee on Pediatric Emergency Medicine and American College of Emergency Physicians Pediatric Committee: Care of children in the emergency department: guidelines for preparedness. *Pediatrics* 107(4):777–781, 2001. Also in: *Ann Emerg Med* 37:389–391, 2001.

19. Gausche-Hill M., Schmitz C., Lewis R.J.: Pediatric preparedness of United States emergency departments: a 2003 survey. *Pediatrics* 120:1229–1237, 2007.

20. Napier J., Knox G.E.: Basic concepts in pediatric patient safety: actions towards a safer health care system. *Clin Pediatr Emerg Med* 7:226–230, 2006.

21. Reason J.: Human error: models and management. *Br Med J* 320:768–770, 2000.

22. Morath J.M.: Patient safety: a view from the top. *Pediatr Clin North Am* 53(6):1053–1065, 2006.

23. Institute of Medicine, Committee on Quality of Health Care in America: *Crossing the Quality Chasm: A New Health System for the 21st Century.* Washington, D.C.: National Academy Press, 2001.

24. Institute of Medicine, Committee on the Work Environment for Nurses and Patient Safety. Keeping Patients Safe: *Transforming the work environment of nurses.* Washington, D.C.: National Academy Press, 2003.

25. Frush K., Krug S., American Academy of Pediatrics Committee on Pediatric Emergency Medicine: Patient safety in the pediatric emergency care setting. *Pediatrics* 120(6):1367–1375, 2007.

26. Barata I.A., Benjamin L.S., Mace S.E., et al.: Pediatric patient safety in the prehospital/emergency department setting. *Pediatr Emerg Care* 23(6):412–418, 2007.

27. Shaw K., Lavelle J., Bonalumi N., et al.: Creating unit-based patient safety walk-rounds in a pediatric emergency department. *Clin Pediatr Emerg Med* 7(4):231–237, 2006.

28. Eppich W.J., Brannen M., Hunt E.A.: Team training: implications for emergency and critical care pediatrics. *Curr Opin Pediatr* 20:255–260, 2008.

29. Salas E., Wilson-Donnelly K.A., Sims D.E., et al.: Teamwork training for patient safety: best practices and guiding principles. In Carayon P (ed.) *Handbook of Human Factors and Ergonomics in Health Care and Patient Safety.* Mahwah, NJ: Erlbaum Associates, 2006.

30. Risser D.T., Rice M.M., Salisbury M.L., et al.: The potential for improved teamwork to reduce medical errors in the emergency department. *Ann Emerg Med* 34:373–383, Sep. 1999.

31. Morey J.C., Simon R., Jay G.D., et al.: Error reduction and performance improvement in the emergency department through formal teamwork training: Evaluation results of the Med Teams project. *Health Ser Res* 37:1553–1581, 2002.

32. American Academy of Pediatrics Committee on Pediatric Emergency Medicine, American College of Emergency Physicians Pediatric Committee, Emergency Nurses Association Pediatric Committee: Guidelines for care of children in the emergency department. *Pediatrics* 124: 1233–1243, Oct. 2009.

33. EMSC National Resource Center. *Facility categorization toolbox.* Children's National Medical Center. Available at: http://www.childrensnational.org/EMSC/PubRes/Facility.aspx (accessed Dec. 5, 2008).

34. Illinois Department of Public Health, Emergency Medical Services for Children: *Facility recognition.* Loyola University Health System. Available at: http://www.luhs.org/depts/emsc/facility.htm (accessed Dec. 5, 2008).

35. California Emergency Medical Services Authority, EMS for Children. *Administration, personnel and policy for the care of pediatric patients in the emergency department.* Available at: http://www.emsa.ca.gov/pubs/pdf/emsa182.pdf (accessed Dec. 5, 2008).

36. Nadzam D., Westergaard F.: Pediatric safety in the emergency department: Identifying risks and preparing to care for child and family. *Journal of Nursing Care Quality* 23:189–194, Jul./Sep. 2008.

37. Institute of Medicine, Committee on the Changing Market, Managed Care, and the Future Viability of Safety Net Providers: *America's Health Care Safety Net: Intact But Endangered.* Washington, D.C.: National Academy Press, 2000.

38. American College of Emergency Physicians, Emergency Medicine Practice Subcommittee on Overcrowding: Information paper. *Emergency department overcrowding.* Dallas, TX: ACEP, Mar. 2004.

39. Margolis L.H., Wagenaar A.C., Molnar L.J.: Use and misuse of automobile child restraint devices. *Am J Dis Child* 146(3): 361–366, 1992.

40. Durbin D.R., Elliott M.R., Winston F.K.: Belt-positioning booster seats and reduction in risk of injury among children in vehicle crashes. *JAMA* 289(21):2835–2840, 2003.

41. Thompson R.S., Rivara F.P., Thompson D.C.: A case-control study of the effectiveness of bicycle safety helmets. *N Engl J Med* 320:1361–1367, May 25, 1989.

42. Gittelman M.A., Durbin D.R.: Injury prevention: is the pediatric emergency department the appropriate place? *Pediatr Emerg Care* 21(7):460–467, 2005.

43. Haddix A., Mallonee S., Waxweiler R., Douglas M.: Cost effectiveness analysis of a smoke alarm giveaway program in Oklahoma City, Oklahoma. *Inj Prev* 7(4):276–281, 2001.

44. Muller A.: Evaluation of the costs and benefits of motorcycle helmet laws. *Am J Public Health* 70(6):586–592, June 1980.

Communication Involving Pediatric Patients and Their Families in the ED and Beyond

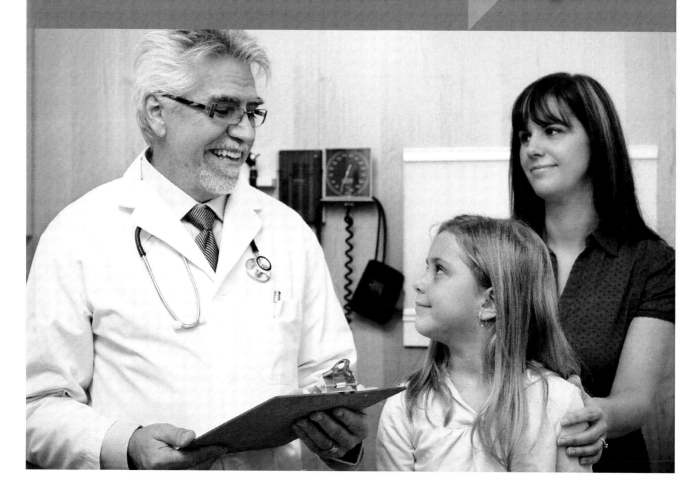

Contributing Editor: Tony Woodward, M.D., M.B.A.,
F.A.A.P., Medical Director, Emergency Services; Chief, Division
of Emergency Medicine at Seattle Children's Hospital

"How can this happen?"

That's a common response to hearing about any adverse health care event, especially by someone not involved in the care giving process. The truth is that communication-related errors happen all too often in every type of health care setting, and the root cause of the errors is frequently as simple as a misunderstood name, as evidenced by the following case study:[1]

"Sydney," a 3-month-old female, was brought to the ED for breathing difficulty by her mother. She was classified as "urgent" for respiratory distress (to be seen by a physician within two hours of initial triage) by the triage nurse at 1:20 p.m. Sydney was registered, and she and her mother were seated in the waiting area. Sydney's mother was told to wait there for placement in a treatment room.

At 2:30 p.m., the primary nurse called Sydney's name. A mother responds—but it is not Sydney's mother. This woman had with her a 3-year-old girl and a 5-year-old boy. The nurse repeated the child's name to the mother, who nodded her head in agreement. In the examination room, the mother was interviewed for historical information by the primary nurse. As the mother spoke only Spanish, her 5-year-old son helped to translate. With this information, the nurse knowingly placed "Cindy," who was still not triaged or registered, in examination room number five. Three-year-old Cindy was misidentified as 3-month-old Sydney, the girl who was triaged more than an hour before.

The ED staff was unaware of the error. A resident completed a history and physical examination for Cindy and documented it on Sydney's chart. Cindy continued to be addressed as "Sydney," and Cindy's Spanish-speaking mother did not acknowledge the difference. The resident and ED attending physician agreed to treat Cindy with a 20 ml/kg of normal saline solution for dehydration; the resident prescribed a 100-ml bolus of normal saline solution based on 4.8-kg weight documented on the wrong chart. The pediatric ED nurse reviewed the physician order and questioned the amount of the fluid bolus as inadequate for the size of the 3-year-old child. The attending, who was fluent in Spanish, examined the child and interviewed her mother. The mother reported that Cindy was recently seen and treated in the ED, but when the attending was unable to find the patient's information in the computer, the attending suspected patient misidentification. The mother verified that her child's name differed from the one on the medical record.

With the misidentification confirmed, Cindy was triaged, registered correctly, and received her own medical record number and chart. Cindy's mother provided consent for treatment at 4:30 p.m., the triage nurse re-evaluated Sydney, who was initially triaged as "urgent." Sydney was upgraded to "emergent" status and placed directly into a patient room to be treated immediately for respiratory distress. Both Cindy and Sydney were later discharged from the ED in stable condition without sequelae.

This incident illustrates the vital importance for standardized expectations and methods of communication, including, but not limited to, the following:

- Team communication
- Patient identification
- Handoffs of care
- Communicating with pediatric patients and their families
- Language challenges

Encouraging Communication Between ED Professionals

The ED is an environment where rapid assessment and intervention is critical, but where care and communication may be fragmented, occur in a discipline-specific silo, and are often interrupted. Because treating patients of many different ages and sizes creates additional opportunities for error in the ED,[2] organizations should design and institute pediatric-specific patient safety policies, procedures, guidelines, and expectations. Optimal staff communication will be integral to successful implementation of those processes.[3–6]

History taking and physical assessment in pediatric patients can be more challenging than it is for adults. Obtaining the history can be a two-or-more-way conversation, sometimes without direct input from the patient, depending on age, medical illness, or developmental maturity. Children are often unable to provide pertinent details of their own medical history or illness, but the detail and accuracy of the medical history may also be imperfect if provided by a parent or other provider—particularly one who is or was not responsible for the day-to-day care of the child.[7] Specifics of complex medical issues may not be offered or heard in acute situations where immediate care is required. Lack of appropriate or accurate information regarding the past medical history, allergies, or medications can be problematic in the acute care of these children. Instructions for subsequent care, an area where we know that what we recommend and prescribe is often not understood or followed, may also fail when delivered through more than one caregiver. Communication with the patient and providers needs to be accomplished in a manner that is easily understood (non-medical terminology and in the caretaker's primary language) and should follow the same guidelines as a medical handoff. These discussions should include "repeat back" or closed-loop communications to ensure understanding of instructions and barrier-free opportunities for questions. And they may also require inclusion of the family/primary care provider to ensure care is instituted as prescribed. The best care delivery in an ED can be negated if the importance of the subsequent management plan is not appreciated or if instructions aren't understood. Verbal communication should be accompanied by written instructions (in the parent's primary language) whenever possible.

A hierarchical structure within the ED medical team may be useful for patient assessment, treatment decisions, overall leadership, and coordination of ED care. Dynamics within the multidisciplinary ED team that "flatten the hierarchy" and reduce discipline-related barriers are critical to effectively prevent errors and enhance quality care for pediatric patients.[7] Although this dynamic of care is often noted in an organization's efforts to develop a culture of safety, the practice of staff communication and information exchange should be emphatically integrated into its ED policies, procedures, and practices. "In the ED, for information to be shared appropriately, it has to be formally recognized by all staff as an integral part of its system of care," says Richard Molteni, M.D., former medical director, Seattle Children's Hospital. "When clinical information management practices are written into policies and procedures that also define roles and responsibilities, all team members are aware of their individual responsibility to communicate among each other to help ensure care consistency and accuracy." Sidebar 2-1, page 24, outlines the core pediatric procedures on which the communication of ED staff rely.

One should also be aware, however, of the dynamic communication challenges in an ED. Several studies have attempted to quantify the amount of interruptions that occur in this environment to help determine the level of risk to safe care. France et al., noted that physicians were interrupted between 5 to 12 times per hour by direct questions or phone calls and that 9% of all direct patient care tasks were interrupted.[8] Woloshynowych et al., studied charge nurse interruptions and noted that ED communications were often chaotic.[9] They noted that the charge R.N. had an average of 100 tasks per hour and that these were interrupted 36% of the time. Spenser and colleagues observed that ED staff spent nearly 90% of their clinical time engaged in communication-related events, with an average of 42 events per staff member per hour.[10] However, 35% of these events were classified as interruptions, with charge nurses and supervisory physicians experiencing more than 20 interruptions per hour. These observations suggest that ED staff and, in particular, frontline clinical managers, have an amazing

amount of information to manage. The presence of frequent interruptions indicates a significant opportunity for improvement. The use of tracking systems, whether via a whiteboard or electronic tracking, may help decrease the need for frequent interruptions of tasks. Although non-verbal communication should not replace face-to-face communication for serious or critical issues, more routine information may be able to be transmitted to more people in a uniform fashion in this manner than by individual conversations. For example, this could include issues about current supply level and inpatient bed status. The whiteboard/electronic tracking system also offers redundancy and more global communication of information than what has been communicated verbally to an individual or set of providers.

Some organizations have moved away from traditional hierarchical or sequential care and patient assessment processes in the ED by adopting a multidisciplinary team approach that revolves around shared information gathering. These have included multidisciplinary primary assessment teams (patient assessed by physician and nursing staff together, rather than the traditional sequential pattern), and nontraditional involvement in care processes (e.g., physician in triage to rapidly process less acute patients, or to start care for those patients who need specified studies or medications that require an order by a licensed provider and traditionally wait until after formal, sequential physician evaluation).

Implementing changes to enhance communication in the ED also necessitates updating to an organization's policies and procedures. Determining what those changes are requires gaining insight from ED staff, patients, and families as well as tracing information—what was transmitted and to whom—in order to evaluate whether particular methods of communication were successful or not. ED staff, referring providers, consultants, admission teams, patients, families, and other providers can help identify gaps in communication and suggest opportunities for improvement. Organizations should also include the input of staff in supporting or partnering departments, such as laboratory, radiology, operating services, pharmacy, and so on in assessing the strengths and weaknesses of ED communication. Safety walk rounds, including ED and hospital administration can be invaluable in seeing the environment in action and giving a clear voice to staff about opportunities for improvement. Ideally these rounds should occur at varied times throughout the 24-hour/365-day service period. In gaining multidisciplinary consensus,

Sidebar 2-1	Care of Children in the Emergency Department

Standardization of care is crucial to optimal ED operations. Standard approaches allow all providers to be oriented to approach and expectations, to understand processes, to identify and justify divergence from standard therapy as well as anticipate and prepare for next steps. Standard process also allows the participant to discuss and educate others involved in the care, including parents and patients. Policies, procedures, guidelines, and protocols for emergency care of children should be developed and implemented, and staff should be educated and monitored accordingly. Hospitals may wish to adopt currently available clinical guidelines and protocols from national or local organizations or use evidence-based information to develop their own.

Communication is critical in the multidisciplinary development of these materials, as well as in the dissemination and implementation of care. Suboptimal communication at any stage of development or implementation of these processes can lead to less than optimal care delivery. ED policies, procedures, guidelines, and protocols should, at a minimum, address the following:

1. Illness and injury triage.

2. Pediatric patient assessment and re-assessment.

3. Documentation of pediatric vital signs, abnormal vital signs, and actions to be taken for abnormal vital signs.

4. Immunization assessment and management of the under-immunized patient.[1]

5. Sedation and analgesia for procedures, including medical imaging.[2,3]

6. Consent (including situations in which a parent is not immediately available).

7. Social and mental health issues.

8. Physical or chemical restraint of patients.

9. Child maltreatment (physical and sexual abuse, sexual assault, and neglect) and domestic violence mandated reporting criteria, requirements, and processes.

10. Death of the child in the ED.[5,6]

11. Do-not-resuscitate orders.

12. Family-centered care,[7–11] including:

  a. Involving families in patient care decision-making and in medication safety processes.

  b. Family presence during all aspects of emergency care, including resuscitation.[11,12]

  c. Education of the patient, family, and regular caregivers.

  d. Discharge planning and instruction.

  e. Bereavement counseling.

13. Communication with patient's medical home or primary health care provider.[13]

14. Medical imaging policies that address age- or weight-appropriate dosing for children receiving studies that impart ionizing radiation, consistent with ALARA (as low as reasonably achievable) principles.[14]

15. All-hazard disaster preparedness plan that addresses the following pediatric issues[15–18]:

  a. A plan that addresses availability of medications, vaccines, equipment, and appropriately trained providers for children in disasters.

  b. A plan that addresses pediatric surge capacity for both injured and noninjured children.

  c. A plan for the decontamination, isolation, and quarantine of families and children of all ages.

  d. A plan to minimize parent-child separation and improved methods for reuniting separated children with their families.

  e. A plan that includes access to specific medical and mental health therapies, as well as social services, for children in the event of a disaster.

  f. A plan that ensures that disaster drills include a pediatric mass casualty incident at least once every two years and that all drills include pediatric patients.

  g. A plan for the care of children with special health care needs.

References

1. American College of Emergency Physicians, Pediatric Committee: Immunization of adults and children in the emergency department. *Ann Emerg Med* 51(5):695, 2008.

2. Cote C.J., Wilson S., and the American Academy of Pediatrics and American Academy of Pediatric Dentistry Work Group on Sedation: Guidelines for monitoring and management of pediatric patients during and after sedation for diagnostic and therapeutic procedures. An update. *Pediatrics* 118(6):2587–2602, 2006.

(Continued on next page)

Sidebar 2-1

Care of Children in the Emergency Department (continued)

3. Mace S., Brown L., and the EMSC Panel (Writing Committee) on Critical Issues in the Sedation of Pediatric Patients in the Emergency Department: Clinical policy: critical issues in the sedation of pediatric patients in the emergency department. *Ann Emerg Med.* 51(4):378–399, 2008.

4. American Academy of Pediatrics, Committee on Pediatric Emergency Medicine: Consent for emergency medical services for children and adolescents. *Pediatrics* 111(3):703–706, 2003.

5. Knapp J., Mulligan-Smith D., and American Academy of Pediatrics, Committee on Pediatric Emergency Medicine: Death of a child in the emergency department. *Pediatrics* 115(5):1432–1437, 2005.

6. Knazik S.R., Gausche-Hill M., Dietrich A.M., et al.: The death of a child in the emergency department. *Ann Emerg Med* 42(4):519–529, 2003.

7. American Academy of Pediatrics, Committee on Hospital Care: Family-centered care and the pediatrician's role. *Pediatrics* 112(3 Pt 1):691–697, 2003.

8. American Academy of Pediatrics, Committee on Emergency Medicine; and American College of Emergency Physicians, Pediatric Committee: Patient- and family-centered care and the role of the emergency physician providing care to a child in the emergency department. *Ann Emerg Med* 48(5):643–645, 2006.

9. American Academy of Pediatrics, Committee on Emergency Medicine; and American College of Emergency Physicians, Pediatric Committee: Patient- and family-centered care and the role of the emergency physician providing care to a child in the emergency department. *Pediatrics* 118(5):2242–2244, 2006.

10. Emergency Nurses Association: *ENA Position Statement: Care of the Pediatric Patient in the Emergency Care Setting.* Des Plaines, IL: Emergency Nurses Association, 2007. Available at: http://www.ena.org/about/position/position/ Pediatric_Patient_in_the_Emergency_Setting_-_ENA_ PS.pdf (accessed Dec. 16, 2008).

11. Guzzetta C.E., Clark A.P., Wright J.L.: Family presence in emergency medical services for children. *Clin Pediatr Emerg Med* 7:15–24, 2006.

12. Emergency Nurses Association: *ENA Position Statement: Family Presence at the Bedside During Invasive Procedures and Cardiopulmonary Resuscitation.* Des Plaines, IL: Emergency Nurses Association, 2005. Available at: http://www.ena.org/about/position/position/ Family_Presence_-_ENA_PS.pdf (accessed Dec. 16, 2008).

13. American Academy of Pediatrics, Medical Home Initiatives for Children With Special Health Care Needs: The medical home. *Pediatrics* 110(1):184–186, 2002.

14. Brody A.S.; Frush D.P.; Huda W.; Brent R.L.; and American Academy of Pediatrics, Section on Radiology: Radiation risk to children from computed tomography. *Pediatrics* 120(3):677–682, 2007.

15. Institute of Medicine, Committee of the Future of Emergency Care in the U.S. Health System: *Emergency Care for Children: Growing Pains.* Washington, D.C.: National Academies Press, 2006.

16. Centers for Bioterrorism Task Force: *Hospital Guidelines for Pediatrics in Disasters.* 2nd ed. New York, N.Y.: New York City Department of Health and Mental Hygiene; 2006. Available at: http://www.nyc.gov/html/doh/ downloads/word/bhpp/bhpp-focus-ped-toolkit.doc (accessed Dec. 15, 2008).

17. American Academy of Pediatrics, Committee on Pediatric Emergency Medicine, Committee on Medical Liability, and Task Force on Terrorism: The pediatrician and disaster preparedness. *Pediatrics* 117(2):560–565, 2006.

18. Markenson D., Reynolds S., and American Academy of Pediatrics, Committee on Pediatric Emergency Medicine and Task Force on Terrorism: The pediatrician and disaster preparedness. *Pediatrics* 117(2):e340– e362, 2006. Available at: http://pediatrics.aappublications.org/cgi/ content/full/117/2/e340 (accessed Dec. 16, 2008).

organizations can move forward with process improvement opportunities likely to have a positive influence on patient care and be embraced by ED providers.

A variation of the traditional safety walk-rounds process, which are usually led by department leadership or hospital administration, are the patient safety walk rounds in the ED at Children's Memorial Hospital in Chicago. The

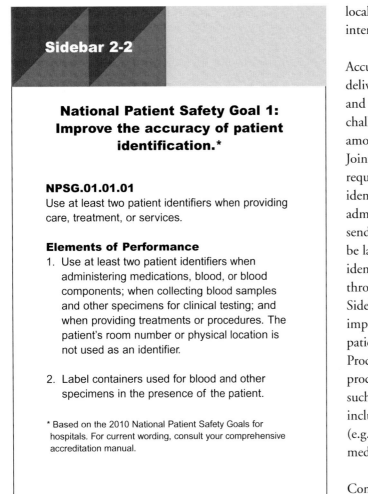

leaders for these rounds are frontline staff, co-led by an ED attending physician and an ED nurse, and are modeled after a process developed by Shaw and colleagues at the Children's Hospital of Philadelphia.[12] The walk rounds leaders, who have been pre-selected and scheduled for this responsibility, enlist the participation of other ED staff who are unaware of this scheduled event in the rounds. This several member ad hoc team gathers data on a variety of issues, ranging from hand washing and infection control practices, to near-misses, and actual safety events that have recently occurred. Both ED staff and patients/families are interviewed regarding their safety concerns. Data gathered is shared at a debriefing session and reported to a multidisciplinary ED safety committee. After an experience of nearly two years, the ED clinical leadership believes that these rounds have helped to promote ED staff use of the hospital's safety event reporting system, and that the perceived culture of safety and the level of staff satisfaction with the ED workplace environment have improved. The walk rounds have also identified a number of meaningful

local priorities for process and safety improvement interventions.

Accuracy of ED patient identification is paramount for delivery of appropriate and safe care. High patient acuity and volume, hectic pace, language and health literacy challenges, multiple providers, and care handoffs are among the factors associated with misidentification. Joint Commission standards and safe patient practices require that organizations use at least two unique patient identifiers. Sending the wrong patient to radiology, administering the wrong drug or drug dose, performing or sending a patient for the wrong procedure, for example, can be largely prevented through care that relies on two unique identifiers. The Joint Commission offers guidelines on this through its National Patient Safety Goal 1, as described in Sidebar 2-2. In addition, use of a time-out process is important for any invasive process in the ED where a patient, procedure, or location could be inaccurate. Procedures in an ED that should have a formal time-out process (communication between all participants and others such as the patient and family involved in the process), include invasive, high risk, or side specific interventions (e.g., arthrocentesis, thoracentesis, lumbar punctures, medical imaging, and others).

Communication through appropriate language is paramount. This can be as simple as using nonmedical language for discussions with families and in discharge planning, to the use of additional personnel to interpret for the patient and family. It is important to consider the functional health literacy of the patient and family when discussing or planning medical issues.[13] One should also note that written and oral health care literacy may not be at the same level. Use of certified interpreters, when primary languages differ, in a face-to-face format, facilitates the most accurate information flow and may maximize patient and family satisfaction.[14–16] Face-to-face certified interpreters enable the conversation to be more than just literal word translations. They may recognize and communicate the important, nonverbal clues or concerns that a patient or family may have. They may also be able to spend noninterview time with the family and identify specific cultural or other concerns or constraints that will impact optimal care delivery. The use of on-site translators is preferred by families over phone interpretation, but the opposite is true for medical professionals. Using family members may limit information obtained if the patient is embarrassed or unwilling to be open and frank with a family member. It may also be problematic when interpretations of medical terms and concepts are not appropriately translated. This is often an issue when the child speaks English and attempts to act as the translator for the non-English speaking parent or caretaker. Translation through non-native, noncertified language speakers (physician, nurses, and students) is discouraged. Although families appreciate the interactions in their primary language, and this conversation is encouraged, important information can be missed by those who are able to speak and understand a second language but are not fluent. Incomplete or inaccurate information obtained during a cross-language conversation can impact care given or expected during or after the evaluation.

Ensuring Effective Communication During Shift Changes

Although few studies have fully documented the safety hazards of "change of shift," it is known that errors occur when staff, including ED staff, fail to communicate clearly to each other about patients in the ED at the time of shift change.[6] The historically hierarchical structure of health care organizations can be a major contributor to the risk of error due to suboptimal communication. One study showed pilots were more likely than surgeons to agree that junior members on the team should be free to question decisions of senior members, suggesting opportunities for improved communication in the surgical disciplines.[17] In high-acuity and high-risk health care settings, and especially in EDs, error-reducing safety nets need to be utilized whenever possible. Barrier-free and effective communication among all members of the ED staff is a key component of that safety net. Communication should be both horizontal and vertical, occurring between all levels and disciplines of care providers for the child. By limiting some from questioning health care professionals with more training or seniority, a safety net that could catch potential errors may be taken away.[18]

"In the ED, overlapping shifts are a serious risk point, especially if communication among staff occurs in discipline-based silos," says Molteni. "This increases hand-off risks, especially when combined with high workload volume and the pressure on staff to generate rapid throughput." In working to avoid the risks caused by lack of staff communication during one of the most critical patient care intervals, many health care organizations are moving toward standardized change-of-shift procedures that involve off-going and on-coming staff and patients. In the ideal situation, all members of the team participate in a face-to-face bedside huddle and utilize the same communication

standards. Although the details of bedside shift reporting need to be customized to an emergency setting and vary from facility to facility, successful implementation results in a real-time exchange of information that improves quality of care, increases accountability, strengthens teamwork, and increases patient safety.[19]

Strategies for effective and error-free handoffs may be found in other high-risk industries where such handoffs occur. Patterson and colleagues observed handoffs in four such high-risk and "high reliability" organizations: the NASA Johnson Space Center, nuclear power plants, and railroad and EMS ambulance dispatch centers.[20] The strategies observed were then analyzed for their potential application to health care. Some of these strategies that might be useful for handoff communications associated with a change of shift, or the physical transfer of a patient to or from the ED include:

- Face-to-face verbal update with interactive questioning
- Topics initiated by incoming and outgoing staff
- The input of staff not being replaced
- Overhear the other team's updates
- Clear transfer of responsibility
- Limit initiation of operator actions during the update
- Limit interruptions during update
- Structured sign-out or checklist

Standardized structures such as SBAR (see page 31 for more information about SBAR) and others can help with a framework for clear and complete handoff communications. Handoffs have many potential errors and pitfalls. Inaccurate, incomplete, insufficient, hurried, or ambiguous information transfer can lead to significant safety implications. Expectations of the information exchange may differ between parties in a handoff. For example, an ED physician may feel the only information that is necessary to convey is that the patient is sick enough to be admitted and is not in extremis, while the inpatient unit physician may feel that more diagnostic and therapeutic information is required to be able to manage the patient in the safest and most appropriate fashion.[21] Time constraints on either side of that discussion can lead to an incomplete or less than optimal handoff and patient care plan. Shendell-Falik, et al., discuss the use of the Appreciative Inquiry technique in improving the patient transfer handoff between the ED and an inpatient unit.[22] Although change of shift or location handoffs offer a clear transfer in responsibility, there are other less obvious handoffs throughout the ED evaluation. These can include staff breaks, transitions with educational providers (resident to resident or attending), transient care providers (consultants, respiratory therapy, radiology team, etc.), patients who are being evaluated by inpatient teams in the ED, patients whose disposition is planned (admission) but still reside in ED after shift change, and boarded patients in the ED whose primary providers may not be clear or present. Multidisciplinary staff huddles are recommended at routine shift changes, as well as whenever challenges are experienced (surge of patients, lack of bed availability, boarding patients, etc.). Indeed, it may be useful for there to be periodic huddles throughout a busy ED shift.

It is also important to recognize that while the handoff may be well done, the actual patient transfer may not immediately occur. When a transfer is delayed, patient reassessment and interim changes should be noted in an updated handoff. It is therefore important for all involved care providers (and arguably the patient and family) to understand who maintains responsibility for the patient. If the participants have changed, a full handoff may need to be repeated for optimal patient safety. When one recognizes the frequency of medical errors in an ED, and that many of these are secondary to failed communication, the need for a standard, formatted, uninterrupted, and complete medical handoff is clear.[23,24]

The 2007 Hospital Survey on Patient Safety Culture conducted by the Agency for Healthcare Research and Quality shows that only 36%–40% of surveyed respondents in hospitals with more than 100 beds indicated that they believed handoffs and transitions generally worked well in their hospital.[25] AHRQ's 2009 release of updated survey results now shows that the "percent positive" score for Handoffs and Transitions scale is 44%; however, it has dropped against the other 11 scales, now among the lowest scoring three scales. Because poor teamwork and communication errors may account for nearly 50% of closed claims involving ED care, and more than 70% of hospital sentinel events, Goal 2 of the Joint Commission's National Patient Safety Goals requires hospitals to "improve the effectiveness of communication among caregivers."

In addition, The Joint Commission requires hospitals to have a process for handoff communication that provides the opportunity for discussion between the giver and receiver of patient information, where such information may include the patient's condition, care, treatment, medications, services, and any recent or anticipated changes to any of these.

Ensuring Effective Communication with Transient or Contracted Staff

ED nurses, physicians, residents, students, technicians, and other team members may be contracted or transient staff who may not be familiar with the organization, its processes and procedures, and/or its terms and abbreviations. As mentioned above, effective communication can be hindered when practitioners relate to one another driven by hierarchy or prior suboptimal experiences. Although perhaps not obvious, a hierarchical barrier may also exist between permanent ED employees and temporary staff. Because of this, it is important to create an atmosphere in which any staff member, regardless of title or employee status, is made aware of expectations and standards and is able to "stop the line," to ask questions and fully participate in care processes. Considering the following questions and providing clear orientation and education regarding practice standards and performance expectations can help leaders and unit managers determine what types of communication challenges and opportunities exist for contracted and transient staff:

- How does orientation take place in your environment? Is it the same for all disciplines? Is the same basic process and logistical information given to all who work in the environment, including contracted employees, transient workers, students, consultants, and others?

- How is communication carried out as part of providing care in your ED?

- Which staff members are involved in the various modes (oral, written, and electronic) of communication?

- What types of communication breakdowns occur that are unique to contracted or transient staff or occur with greater frequency when staffing with these providers? Is the breakdown in communication a direct effect of these staff not knowing your organization's policies and procedures? Is it that the staff member does not know where to get needed information or is not asking for assistance? Is it a breakdown in the system itself? Is it a misinterpretation of a policy or expectation?

After investigating and identifying barriers to communication among contracted and transient staff, your organization can move to determine which ones pose the greatest risk to patients and which ones are most likely to occur. Your ED can then begin making improvements that will result in more effective communication with temporary or contracted staff. Seeking feedback from these staff members and from frontline staff who regularly work side-by-side will help to ensure that improvement efforts have their intended benefit. In Sidebar 2-3, right, strategies for improving communication with contracted and transient staff are further discussed.

Improving Transfer Communication

A pediatric patient can be cared for in many areas during one hospital stay, from the ED to the operating room, intensive care unit, step-down unit, and medical/surgical unit. In this process, staff are not simply moving patients but transferring critical historical and current information, care plans with contingency suggestions, and medical responsibility for a patient. These handoffs can also include transfers to different hospitals and ambulatory care providers.

"Because staff members hand off information about patients so often, they may not realize handoff communication is a high-risk process," says Grena Porto, R.N., a patient safety expert who sits on the Joint Commission's Sentinel Event Advisory Committee. "If staff members do not allocate enough time to a hand off, one or the other staff member may not get a complete picture of the patient's situation and important information can be lost. This is a common cause of error,"[26] and an important point to consider. Most hospital care systems do not allot time in the transition process for a full and complete handoff. The incoming team and the outgoing team may start and end shifts at the same time, so the incentive is to have a quick handoff to allow one group to start their work and the other to leave for the day. Patients currently undergoing care may be caught in the middle of a cursory handoff and an inadequate information transfer that affects the care they ultimately receive.

Ensuring the effective transfer of medical information depends on a standardized approach to the process, one that includes a focused, standardized, uninterrupted presentation, and an opportunity for staff to discuss the case, ask, and respond to questions. The following five strategies are designed to strengthen handoff communication[27]:

1. Use clear language. Avoid unclear or potentially confusing terms (such as, "she's a little unstable," "he's doing fine," or "she's lethargic"). Identify the patient exactly and define the terms you're using. Don't use abbreviations or jargon that could be misinterpreted.

2. Incorporate effective communication techniques. Limit interruptions, focus on the information being exchanged, and allocate sufficient time to this important task. Implement read-back or check-back techniques to make sure there is a common understanding about

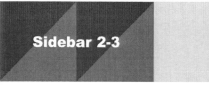

Sidebar 2-3

Strategies for Improving Communication with Contracted and Transient Staff

Talk the Talk
Help staff express themselves by discussing any jargon or terms commonly used in your ED or by different disciplines or units. Be sure to use specific examples. In addition, it may be helpful to review methods of phrasing questions and responses in a concise, yet nonconfrontational manner. Also, provide detailed examples of ways to verify spoken or telephone communications that are difficult to understand. The idea is to focus on improving care for pediatric patients by preventing miscommunication.

Seek Help from Risk Managers
Risk managers are in an excellent position in your organization to know the underlying causes of adverse events and near misses. Ask your organization's risk manager to flag data that show any communication problems associated with the use of contracted staff and provide ideas for how to improve processes.

expectations. Encourage interactive questioning to allow for better information absorption. Keep the report patient-centered and avoid irrelevant details. Involve the parents and family in the communications whenever possible.

3. Standardize shift-to-shift and unit-to-unit reporting. A consistent format increases the amount of information staff members accurately record and recall and improves their ability to plan patient care. Organize the data with a sign-out checklist, a script, or an "at a glance" status display. Checklists have demonstrated effectiveness in reducing errors in other industries and have been observed to reduce error in other high-risk healthcare settings, such as the operating room and the intensive care unit.[28] Provide cues of important information to pass on that is otherwise likely to be forgotten in the chaos of shift or unit changes. Keep the report concise and accurate. What you include in handoff communications varies by setting and discipline, but can include a summary of the patient's current medical status, resuscitation status,

recent lab values, allergies, a problem list, a current medication list, and a to-do list for the covering physician or nurse. Get input from front-line staff to identify what should be included in the report. At Ohio State University Hospital, residents use "MD Notes," a computerized sign-out program, to enter patient information and action plans for care for covering physicians. The process concludes with a face-to-face meeting. Organizations can also consider using the Situation-Background-Assessment-Recommendation (SBAR) technique to standardize communications explained in Sidebar 2-4 on page 31.

4. Establish effective handoffs between care settings. The transition between settings of care (such as from the hospital to home) can be unpredictable. To prevent problems, communicate with the primary care physician when a patient is admitted and provide updates whenever the patient's status changes significantly. On discharge, provide the patient's family and his or her medical home with information about discharge diagnoses, medications, and results of procedures and labs. As patients and/or their families may have misunderstood or do not recall home-going care instructions, a simple follow-up call to the patient or patient's family by a physician, nurse, or pharmacist can prevent many post-discharge errors.

5. Use technology to your advantage. Communication systems that transmit information across settings and care providers can bring consistency and coordination to care practices. For example, automated medication reconciliation and problem lists between settings of care, such as shared access of patient records between physician office practices and hospitals, helps to streamline procedures, such as medication reconciliation, during admissions and discharges. Likewise, access to immunization registries may assist providers caring for pediatric patients in the ED. Electronic medical records can facilitate transitions by providing consistent, accessible information about patients and their care. Staff members should be able to readily access essential components of care, such as whether a newly ordered medication was administered, whether labs were done, or if a do-not-resuscitate order is in place. Keep electronic approaches interactive and effective by making time to answer questions or provide updates before signing off responsibility.

It is important that ED staff organize and coordinate handoff and discharge procedures around the specific illness of the child, especially for those with chronic illnesses.[29]

After communicating test results, medication information and discharge instructions to the patient's family and PCP and/or sub-specialty care physician, ED staff should follow up with the patient/family to confirm that they also perceive that the patient's condition has improved and that they fully understand and will be able to adhere to planned outpatient therapy.

Strengthening Initial (Pre-Admission or Pre-Arrival) Communication

Developing a strong relationship with primary and specialty care providers is important in gaining essential medical information prior to patient arrival and in a timely manner after a pediatric patient arrives in the ED. This communication is especially important when caring for children who are medically complex. At pre-admission or pre-arrival, ED staff need as much information as possible about an arriving patient in order to effectively prepare the staff and environment for the patient's needs. This communication should occur in a standard fashion that mirrors a unit handoff, with clinical information presented in a standard fashion (chief complaint, pertinent medical history, significant past medical history, vital signs, pertinent physical examination, ancillary studies, interventions, and response to those interventions). This is a critical handoff, often involving acutely ill children, which may take place between providers who may not know each other, the capabilities of either system, or on occasion, the complete information regarding the ill patient. The Emergency Information Form jointly developed by the American Academy of Pediatrics and the American College of Emergency Physicians in their 1999 policy statement, "Emergency Preparedness for Children With Special Health Care Needs," can be a useful adjunct in this situation.[29] See Table 7-1 on page 120.

A complete, timely, and accurate medication history is a critical component of a thorough patient history. Asking the right questions is a crucial step in the process of properly detailing a patient's full medication history. Does the patient have an ongoing medical issue? What drugs is the patient already taking? This information should be documented in a standard fashion and available to all members of the acute care team.

At Seattle Children's Hospital, a 24/7 nurse-staffed ED communication center takes information from referring providers and documents this information on the patient's actual chart and also posts the pre-arrival information on an electronic tracking system, visible to providers throughout the institution. This process allows the information to be

Defining the Situation-Background-Assessment-Recommendation (SBAR) Technique to Standardize Communication

Physicians and nurses communicate and think differently because they are educated differently. Nurses tend to use a narrative approach when communicating, while physicians can be more focused when attempting to determine and then fix a problem.[1] Although neither method is necessarily superior to the other, these and other communication differences may cause confusion. Other factors that contribute to miscommunication between physicians and nurses include the following[1]:

- Gender
- Culture
- Multitasking
- Short-term memory limitations
- Fatigue
- Stress
- A fast-paced environment with multiple simultaneous demands, distractions, and interruptions
- Intimidation due to the hierarchical nature of health care organizations

Hierarchy or authority gradients can be a root cause of medical error in health care settings.[2] Authority gradients were first noted as a safety concern in the aviation industry. The presence of a perceived difference in experience, rank, or authority, such as between a co-pilot and a pilot, or between a resident and attending physician, or a nurse and a physician, could cause the team member with less experience (or lower rank) to be reluctant to express their concern about a procedure, order, or decision that they fear will harm the patient.

Authority gradients may be especially prevalent in academic settings but can occur in any ED. Team training, including the use of critical language, has worked to reduce this phenomenon in aviation and is a strategy that may prove to be effective in healthcare.

The Situation–Background–Assessment–Recommendation (SBAR) technique requires the following types of information to be transferred between caregivers[1]:

- Situation—What is going on with the patient?
- Background—What is the clinical background or context?
- Assessment—What do I think the problem is?
- Recommendation—What would I do to correct it?

SBAR was originally used by the military for nuclear submarines.[3] Michael Leonard and colleagues Doug Bonacum and Suzanne Graham developed a health care version of this technique to aid physician-nurse communication.[3]

References

1. Joint Commission Resources: The SBAR technique: Improves communication, enhances patient safety. *Patient Safety* 5:1–2, 8, Feb. 2006.
2. Cosby K.S., Croskerry P.: Profiles in patient safety: authority gradients in medical error. *Academic Emergency Medicine* 11:1341–1345, 2004.
3. Zimmerman P.G.: Cutting-edge discussions of management, policy, and program issues in emergency care. *J Emerg Nurs* 32:267–268, Jun. 2006.

gathered in a standard fashion and follow the patient throughout the ED evaluation and, if necessary, admission to the hospital. Including this information as part of the medical record is vital in ensuring that critical information accompanies the patient, not an individual or singular group of providers. Having patient-specific information gathered in a central location prevents issues with potential loss or nontransmission of this information when a single provider collects the data, documents it in a nonstandard way and potentially cares for a patient assuming all are aware of the same information. Key medical information called in by phone and written down on a piece of paper by a staff member can easily be lost or not communicated to the nurse or physician caring for the patient, so this should

be avoided. Whenever possible, parents should be asked to *bring* the child's medication and medical history with them when referred directly from a physician's office.

Although a parent or family member of a pediatric patient arriving in the ED serves as a primary and initial source of this important information, organizations must establish effective paths of communication with primary and specialty care providers and other health care professionals and systems in the community to ensure access to appropriate and accurate information. Going beyond building relationships with PCPs, organizations must develop clear and reliable systems of information delivery. This can include access to radiographic or laboratory studies as well as pertinent medical records. For instance, reliable systems such as computerized patient information systems or Internet-based systems that are networked with other health care providers in the community including local pharmacies would be a great step forward in making critical information available to ED providers. Shapiro et al., nicely describe the opportunities and impact one could make with improved communication between health care systems.[30] They noted that in one ED, 25% of the patients with greater than one ED visit in a year had had care delivered in another health care system. This subset accounted for 19% of the total ED visits for that year.

If each health care provider is not aware of what is happening with a patient from all perspectives, a provider could begin a new therapy or augment an existing one, which could lead to redundancy, increased risk and exposures, or increased cost and patient safety issues.[31] In the ED, electronic medical records can provide clinicians with more complete information in a timely fashion, and, logically, could provide better pediatric patient care.

Although electronic and Internet-based systems with the ability to rapidly retrieve many or all aspects of a patient's medical record are already in place in many institutions around the country, it is personal communication that ultimately determines their effectiveness in reducing the risks of medical error. Crew resource management (CRM), a communication model developed in the aviation industry and incorporated into various components of the health care system, emphasizes the role of human factors in high-stress, high-risk environments such as the ED. The CRM model relies on a system of cross-monitoring by members of the health care team and, while also recognizing hierarchical structures of the department, professes that any member of the team—regardless of his or her level in the organization—must feel comfortable raising questions or concerns without hesitation.[32] (*See* Sidebar 2-5, page 33 to learn how CRM can be used in health care.)

Communication must also be encouraged when errors or near misses occur. It is clear that families want and expect to know if an error has occurred that may or will affect the patient.[33] It is not as clear that they want the same level of disclosure for near misses. It is important, however, that the medical system and health care teams develop a culture of blame-free and open communication for both of these areas of concern. This allows errors and near misses to be acknowledged and evaluated in a systematic fashion. Awareness will also allow trends to be determined and opportunities for improvement at a system level to be

investigated. An interesting study, by Wu et al., first published in 1991, found that 76% of house officers had not disclosed a serious error when they had been involved.[34] Although providers may feel that disclosure increases the risk of medical liability, this has not been shown to be true. This may be especially important in an ED where there has often not been a relationship established between the providers (and sometimes the institution) and the patient/family.

Insisting on Medication Reconciliation

Medication reconciliation is the process of comparing what medication the patient is taking at the time of admission or entry to a new setting or level of care, with what the organization is providing (admission, ED medication, or discharge orders) to avoid errors such as redundancy, conflict, or unintentional omissions. Like medical histories, when a patient's medication information is unreliably communicated to or processed by ED care providers, it can negatively impact patient care. For example, a staff member who obtains verbal pre-arrival information from the patient's PCP may not have full information and may communicate the limited information incorrectly to ED staff. Depending on the circumstance, there could be a number of specialists managing different components of a child's care. Pertinent information may be unavailable because it exists in a shadow chart, a parallel medical record containing confidential information, or with an individual provider. This information is now unavailable to the ED staff. Cultural and language barriers can also impact the communication of medication information. Not only is the concept of medication reconciliation important, the communication that must occur for a system to be optimal is crucial. At Seattle Children's Hospital, medication reconciliation is a process that involves several disciplines. Medication technicians (pharmacy techs) are stationed in the ED 24 hours a day. They have the responsibility of interviewing every family to determine current medications. These data are entered into a central information system and reconciled by the treating physician team. Also included in this reconciliation are all medications previously entered and reconciled if the patient has been cared for in the hospital system in the past. This list is reviewed prior to medication administration in the ED as well as when prescriptions are written (electronically) and added to the list at time of discharge. Conflicts are noted when they occur and are communicated by staff to each other and the patient/family. This information is then communicated to the next level of providers, whether an inpatient team or an outpatient provider, as well as given

| Sidebar 2-5 | **Applying Crew Resource Management (CRM) to Health Care** |

What Is CRM, and How Is It Relevant to Health Care?

From several workshops in 1979 and 1980, the aviation industry concluded that failures of collaborative interaction and teamwork were responsible for 70% of airline crashes examined.[1] In response to these findings, airline companies began developing training programs for cockpit personnel, originally known as *cockpit resource management,* which focused on flight personnel in cockpit simulators.[2] These programs subsequently expanded to include the entire flight crew, maintenance crews, and air traffic controllers, and became known as *CRM.* The CRM model focuses on the safety, efficiency, and morale of people working together. Although no definitive study has correlated CRM training with enhanced airline flight safety, the aviation industry accepts this practice at face value, and CRM training is an international requirement for all aviation employees.[3,4] CRM has moved aviation training beyond the limited focus of technical flying to broader dimensions of human factors engineering, fatigue and stress management, effective communication, shared awareness, and teamwork. In surveys, airline crew members consistently cite CRM training as relevant, useful, and effective in changing attitudes and behaviors to improve safety.[5]

Cross-sectional surveys have suggested that safety-related behaviors applied and studied extensively in aviation may also be relevant in health care.[5] Helmreich and Merritt have proposed a translation of teamwork behaviors from aviation to health care by the application of "countermeasures"— briefings, debriefings, standardized communication language and processes, workload distribution, fatigue management, inquiry, graded assertiveness, contingency planning, and conflict resolution—introduced in CRM training.[6] CRM applications in a simulated work environment have been applied in operating rooms, intensive care units, labor and delivery units for neonatal resuscitation, and hospital emergency departments.[7–10] CRM training has been undertaken for multiple medical disciplines in large health systems.[11,12]

Of course, ED teams are clearly somewhat different than cockpit teams. Constantly changing members (e.g., temporary staff, rotating residents, consultants) complicates team communication processes. Also within these ad hoc teams, there exist separate hierarchies of power and training, adding further to complexity. Finally, ED team members may possess varying levels of experience, particularly in academic centers. Team training may prove to be useful in teaching core components of teamwork, including team leadership, mutual performance monitoring and back-up behaviors by team members, and team attitude or orientation. Central to effective teamwork is the ability for members to communicate in a manner that allows the development of a common understanding about the situation at hand, a shared mental model. This skill may also be taught in team training.

Adapted from Dunn E.J., et al.: Team training: Applying crew resource management in the Veterans Health Administration. *Jt Comm J Qual Patient Saf* 33(6):317–325, Jun. 2007; and Eppich W.J., Brannen M., Hunt E.A.: Team training: implications for emergency and critical care pediatrics. *Current Opinion in Pediatrics* 20:255–260, 2008.

References

1. Pizzi L., Goldfarb N., Nash D.: *Crew Resource Management and its Application in Medicine.* San Francisco: UCSF-Stanford Evidence Based Practice Center, 2001, pp. 501–509.

2. Weiner E., Kanki B., Helmreich R.: *Cockpit Resource Management.* San Diego: Academic Press, 1993.

3. Helmreich R., Wilhelm J.: Outcomes of crew resource management training. *International Journal of Aviation Psychology* 1(4):287–300, 1991.

4. Salas E., Burke C., Bowers C.: Team training in the skies: Does crew resource management (CRM) really work? *Human Factors* 41:641–674, Winter 1999.

5. Sexton J., Thomas E., Helmreich R.: Error, stress, and teamwork in medicine and aviation: Cross sectional surveys. *BMJ* 320:745–749, Mar. 2000.

6. Helmreich R.L., Merritt A.C.: *Culture at Work in Aviation and Medicine: National, Organizational and Professional Influences.* Brookfield, VT: Ashgate Publishing, 2001.

7. Risser D., Rice M.M., Salisbury M.L., et al.: The potential for improved teamwork to reduce medical errors in the emergency department. *Ann Emerg Med* 34:373–383, Sep. 1999.

8. Howard S., Gaba D.M., Fish K.J., et al.: Anesthesia crisis resource management training: Teaching anesthesiologists to handle critical incidents. *Aviat Space Environ Med* 63:763–770, Sep. 1992.

9. Halamek L.P., Kaegi D.M., Gaba D.M., et al.: Time for a new paradigm in pediatric medicine education: Teaching neonatal resuscitation in a simulate delivery room environment. *Pediatrics* 106:E45, Oct. 2000.

10. Baker D., Gustafson S., Beaubren J.M., et al.: Medical team training programs in health care. *Advances in Patient Safety* 4:253–267, 2005. http://www.ahrq.gov/downloads/pub/advances/vol4/Baker.pdf (accessed Jul. 17, 2009).

11. Grogan E.L., Stiles R.A., France D.J., et al.: The impact of aviation-based teamwork training on the attitudes of health-care professionals. *J Am Coll Surg* 199:843–848, Dec. 2004.

12. Leonard M., Graham S., Bonacum D.: The human factor: The critical importance of effective teamwork and communication in providing safe care. *Qual Saf Health Care* 13:185–190, Oct. 2004.

to the family as part of the discharge materials. Additional information about medication reconciliation can be found in Chapter 4.

Encouraging Families to Carry Medical Information

As medication reconciliation and effective ED treatment depend on accurate information provided on a patient's arrival, organizations should encourage families to make a practice of carrying the medical information of their children with them at all times. Rather than relying solely on the investigative work of ED staff or locally available medical records, the parents and caregivers can have important aspects of their child's medical history accessible when an emergency situation occurs. This can be especially helpful for children with complex health conditions who may be receiving care from several specialists simultaneously. The AAP/ACEP "Emergency Information Form" can be very helpful in this situation.[29] Although it may not seem important, staff awareness of even the smallest detail could potentially be crucial in the care of the medically complex pediatric patient.

Although it is not practical to carry a full medical record at all times, there are alternatives. A simple solution for parents is to develop a one-page summary of a child's medical history. This single piece of paper could be carried in a purse or wallet and kept with the parent or caregiver at all times. The information should be complete, compiled as lists rather than as sentences or paragraphs. Names and phone numbers of providers as well as photocopies of any special tests (EKGs, etc.), if applicable, could be attached to this document. ED staff should be sure this information is captured in a reliable manner so that the condition(s) or medication listed can be updated but does not have to be recreated at each visit.

The Internet provides another option for the maintenance of family medical records. Many companies have developed Web sites designed for recording medical information that can be reached from any computer with Internet access such as www.webmd.com and www.health-minder.com. Some of these companies even have options for printing a summary of the information that parents can carry with them. Some of the sites are designed to allow doctors access to the information in emergencies. One excellent example is the EMSC-funded project in the State of Minnesota for children with congenital heart disease. The Minnesota Emergency Medical Services for Children Information System (MEMSCIS) provides a secure and HIPAA-compliant, Internet-based repository (http://www.emscmn.org/Healthcare

Professionals/specialhealth.asp) for key clinical information regarding medically complex children that can be accessed 24/7 by emergency care providers.

The increasing popularity of digital, handheld personal computers and devices makes electronic maintenance of a child's medical record quite practical. A wide variety of software for these personal data assistants is commonly available; many programs can be purchased via the Internet.

Although community pediatricians and primary care providers can help parents develop a customized checklist or toolkit to work from in building a medical brief, Sidebar 2-6, page 35, outlines the primary information that parents should include. In addition, family and patient medical history forms may be used by patients and parents of patients to include important medical history and medication information as a printout, downloaded onto a PDA, or even e-mailed to a personal e-mail account that would be accessible from any internet-ready computer. Various forms are available through organization Web sites, including the following:

- The American Academy of Pediatrics http://www.medicalhomeinfo.org/tools/ care_notebook.html

- The American Medical Association http://www.ama-assn.org/ama/pub/physician-resources/medical-science/genetics-molecular-medicine/family-history.shtml

- The Centers for Disease Control and Prevention http://www.cdc.gov/genomics/public/famhist.htm

Parents should keep and maintain a more extensive medical record file on their child at home. With information that ranges from birth certificates to the names of pharmacies that have filled prescriptions, this home file can prove invaluable to a child's future medical treatment. For children with chronic illnesses, keeping a journal of important events, tests, medications and dosages, appointments, ED or urgent care visits, and so on, may prove to be beneficial in emergency situations. It has even been recommended that a copy of the child's medical summary be kept on refrigerators at home so it may be easily located by EMS responders. This information should also be duplicated and kept in a secure, waterproof container for disaster scenarios and should be part of a family disaster readiness kit.

Gaining the Trust of Patients and Families

Obtaining important medical information from pediatric patients and their families also depends on gaining their trust. Practitioners who can connect with patients at the

| **Sidebar 2-6** | **Making a Child's Medical Information Accessible to ED Staff** |

To help certain emergency staff know the details of a pediatric patient's medical history, parents or caregivers should carry the following important information with them at all times.

Immunizations, medical problems, and care providers: Parents should always keep a record of their children's childhood immunizations and a list of every current and past medical problem. This should include chronic diseases (such as asthma, cancer, diabetes, HIV/AIDS, and others), as well as a list of illnesses, hospitalizations, surgeries, and the names and contact information for all of the child's medical providers.

Current medications and allergies: Vitally important as well is a comprehensive list of any medication a child is currently taking, and how much and how often the child takes it. Medicines such as anticoagulants, diuretics, steroids and other anti-inflammatory agents, anti-epileptics, and other agents can all influence your child's treatment. Also include any alternative, herbal, or over-the-counter medications or vitamins. Equally important is a list of all medical allergies. Some children have very serious allergies to common medications or medical equipment. Essential allergies to list include latex, medications (such as antibiotics, aspirin, heparin, penicillin, sulfa-based drugs) and contrast dyes, significant food allergies, as well as any other medical allergy. Additionally, parents should try to describe, in writing, any allergic reaction a child has experienced—such as itching, rash, urticaria, anaphylaxis, swelling, or respiratory distress.

Family medical history: Include all of your family's medical problems, especially parents' (yours) and siblings', but also information about other family members that may also be pertinent (a family history of cancer, for example).

Phone numbers: Have phone numbers for family members and all of your child's health care providers. The ED can contact any pertinent provider for additional medical history and post-care follow-up.

Medical data: Patients with uncommon chronic diseases should have information available for the ED provider, who may not be aware of their specific medical history. These conditions could range from a routine disease process such as asthma to a more complex metabolic illness. Some children may need to have copies of any abnormal or recent laboratory tests or examinations. Those with heart disease should try to have a copy of their most recent ECG and results of heart catheterization (if they have had one), echocardiogram, or stress tests. The parent of a child with anemia or HIV should try to list their child's most recent blood counts. Those with asthma could have their peak flow measurements available as well. Similarly, children with liver or kidney disease need their most recent liver or kidney test results. A clinical summary letter, written by the child's subspecialty care provider, can be requested by families for the purpose of informing acute care providers in the ED setting.

Care plans: Equally important is access to specific care plans. For patients with unusual, complex, or fragile medical conditions, access to a care plan developed by the PCP and/or specialist can be life-saving. For example, while the treatment of some patients with an underlying metabolic disease can be straightforward, not knowing the nuances of the disease or patient-specific fluid and electrolyte, glucose, or hormone therapy requirements can delay appropriate care. As care plans and treatment guidelines describe standard therapy and expectations for medical providers, a patient care plan can do the same for the medically complex child who presents for care to an institution where ED staff may not have the experience managing a child with special health care needs. When families have made difficult decisions to limit extraordinary care or resuscitation, this information should be immediately available to the ED team.

Adapted from Family-Friendly-Fund Home Page, http://family-friendly-fun.com/health/medical-records.htm (accessed June 4, 2009).

outset enhance the environment of care and open lines of communication that can be instrumental in determining effective treatment. The initial medical interview of the patient and family will be the primary opportunity to assess the presence of limited health literacy, the need for language translation, and concerns for cultural competency.

As this important information is gathered from the patient and family, it is likewise important to ensure that effective bidirectional communication has been achieved. With effective communication achieved, this also becomes a great opportunity to gain patient/family trust, demonstrate family-centered care practices, and a pro-active concern

---

Sidebar 2-7

Considerations While Communicating With a Patient's Family

Pediatric patients presenting to the ED should be interviewed whenever possible to try to determine their symptoms and the underlying problem. When children cannot speak for themselves, they rely on their parents to convey information about their condition that may complicate a situation when a parent attempts to explain a problem. Parents may not always have an objective view of their child's issues. Although most will be accurate and clear about medical issues and degree of illness, others may be unable to do so due to limited health literacy, or simply secondary to fatigue, stress, other competing concerns, or the patient's acuity. Parents may

- see their child as being more or less ill than they appear to the medical provider and the parent may not agree with the acuity assessment of the ED staff. Although this can be challenging, it is also an opportunity for the ED staff to reevaluate their initial assessment, if the people who know the child best think that the evaluation may be incomplete or misdirected. This practice may prove to be especially useful when caring for children with special health care needs.

- have preconceived ideas of what the condition might be and insist on medication or tests that are either unnecessary or inappropriate for the child's condition,

or refuse therapy deemed to be vital for the evaluation and care of the patient. For the extremes of these interactions, including others who have established relationships with the patient and family (PCP, specialist, religious leader, or extended family members) may be helpful in negotiating a safe and effective plan of action.

- not know what is wrong, possibly triggering less experienced staff to conduct more tests that expose the child to more diagnostic error (e.g., false positive test results) or potential adverse side effects of diagnostic tests (e.g., radiation from medical imaging).

It is equally important that providers carefully listen to families as they provide patient information. If families become frustrated with our interactions, it may be that they perceive we aren't hearing what they are telling us, perhaps as we try to fit the patient into our initial disease categorization or assessment of acuity level. This can be especially challenging when patients return to the ED several times. As providers, we may have the tendency to dismiss these return visits as secondary to patient/parental over concern or anxiety, but, in reality, we need to step back and potentially broaden our differential diagnosis and consider what we may be missing that requires additional visits to the ED.

Adapted from Frush, Karen, B.S.N., M.D., Chief Patient Safety Officer, Duke University Health System. Telephone interview on June 15, 2007.

---

for patient safety. Communicating with children, however—especially those who find themselves in the ED battling an illness—can be even more challenging than communicating with adults. Children may be fatigued, scared, confused, feeling ill, or experiencing pain, and may be unable to communicate with ED staff, further complicating the ED experience for pediatric patients and their families/providers.

The pediatric interview, for example, is more complicated than the traditional adult patient medical interview because it should be conducted with at least one additional party—a home care provider, and often several other interested and involved family members.[35] Unfortunately, this frequently results in children being left out of the interview process.[36] Depending on the age of the patient, ED clinicians should determine how much of the questioning and discussion should be directed to the patient. As much as possible, ED clinicians should involve younger patients in the interview process. For adolescent patients, it may be important to conduct aspects of the interview (and the exam with an

appropriate chaperone as indicated) primarily with the patient. For this to occur, it is perfectly acceptable to ask the parent to step out. One can then reassure the patient regarding confidentiality and ask about sexual activity and substance abuse. This is also an opportunity to ask about other potential sources of abuse including physical, sexual, and/or emotional abuse. This assessment should be performed in a nonjudgmental manner.

Studies have shown that actively involving children in their own health care greatly improves both parent and child satisfaction with the medical interview, increases children's knowledge of their medication, and improves the overall functional status of children.[36] Perhaps just as important is the concept of family-centered care, recognizing the importance of the family unit in support of a child with a medical illness.[37] Sidebar 2-7, above, discusses additional considerations regarding communication with patients and families.

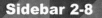

Sidebar 2-8

Communication Enhancers

Don't omit pleasantries—build rapport, say hello. Make eye contact with each member of the patient/family group and shake hands as appropriate (acknowledging cultural differences where needed). Use positive body language to help demonstrate your commitment to listening and teamwork with the family regarding diagnosis and care.

Introduce yourself by name and title.

Refer to the parent and patient by name, not role (i.e., "Ms. Smith" rather than "Mom," "Jake" rather than "your child, he or she")

Don't appear rushed, even if you are.

Keep conversations on track. "I know you are concerned about ... but I would like to focus on ..."

Relate to patients. Be sincere with your eyes. If you need to document on paper or on a computer during the discussion, acknowledge and explain that fact to the family. ("I will be writing/typing while we talk. This is important for me to ensure that I don't miss any of the important information we discuss.")

One option is to organize the interview using the BATHE technique. While this may not be the appropriate or complete technique for all patients and families (especially complex patients or difficult interactions), it provides a reasonable starting point for the interview process:

B = Background: "Tell me what has been happening."

A = Affect: "How do you feel about that?"

T = Trouble: "What is upsetting you most about it?"

H = Handling: "How are you handling the situation?"

E = Empathy: "That must have been difficult for you."

Adapted from Belzer E.: Patient relations: Improving patient communication in no time. *Fam Pract Manage* 6–5, 1999.

Sidebar 2-9

Label the Emotion and Generalize It

Practitioner: "You seem scared or afraid about the needle."

Practitioner: "Are you worried that it is going to hurt?"

Practitioner: "I know this is scary. Lots of kids feel nervous about shots. Your blood won't leak out, but it might sting for a few seconds. How about we put a bandage on it afterwards. Will that work?"

One should, however, be careful with questions that might lead to an answer that is not acceptable. For example, one should not ask the patient if it is OK to proceed (with a shot for instance), unless the patient really has that control (to have the shot or not). If they don't, the question should be framed in a different manner and address some aspect of the care where control can be shifted to the patient ("After we give you the medicine, you can have a bandage if you like. It can be a plain bandaid or one of our special cartoon character bandages— which one would you like?").

Adapted from O'Neill K.A.: Kids speak: Effective communication with the school-aged/adolescent patient. *Pediatr Emerg Care* 18(2):137–138, 2002.

Time constraints are a constant challenge in the ED. Effective communication with a pediatric patient and their family requires striking a balance between being a good listener (to the patient and the family) and efficiently getting accurate information that enables decisions to be made regarding the etiology of presentation and appropriate management. Sidebar 2-8, above, offers some quick, simple suggestions to increase the efficiency of the interview process.

Talking to children about their emotions allows them to label their feelings and better cope with their illness. In the interview process, practitioners can explore a patient's and/or parent's emotions by asking questions in a general or universal way that leads toward drawing more concrete information. They might also begin with depicting a particular scenario that has a focus in mind. For example, a practitioner wanting to find out if a boy has had difficulty making friends at school might start off by asking, "How do you like recess time at school?" The conversation can continue with follow-up questions such as, "Do you get to play games? Do you have any special friends that you play with?"[13] Although perhaps not applicable to all patients, parents, or situations, these general or universal questions can be used again in the treatment of a child, as described in Sidebar 2-9, above.

Choosing questions carefully and engaging in conversation that allows the patient to feel comfortable in telling his or her story—perhaps followed by the parent's version of the story—enables clinicians to draw information that can be immediately put to use in the care process. Recognizing the patient's feelings can be therapeutic for the patient and family alike. Family-centered care is predicated on the fact that the child is part of a larger unit. Recognition of that fact can help us design an optimal process for care in our ED environment and have a powerful and positive impact on the ED environment of care.

References

1. O'Neill K.A., Shinn D., Starr K.T., et al.: Patient misidentification in a pediatric emergency department: Patient safety and legal perspectives. *Pediatric Emergency Care* 20(7):487–491, 2004.

2. Kozer E., Scolnic D., Macpherson A., et al.: Variables associated with medication errors in pediatric emergency medicine. *Pediatrics* 110:737–742, 2002.

3. Institute of Medicine Committee on the Future of Emergency Care in the United States Health System: *Emergency care for children: growing pains.* Washington, D.C.: National Academy Press, 2006.

4. Institute of Medicine Committee on the Future of Emergency Care in the United States Health System: *Emergency medical services: at the crossroads.* Washington, D.C.: National Academy Press, 2006.

5. Institute of Medicine Committee on the Future of Emergency Care in the United States Health System: *Hospital-based emergency care: at the breaking point.* Washington, D.C.: National Academy Press, 2006.

6. Frush K., Krug S.E., Committee on Pediatric Emergency Medicine, American Academy of Pediatrics: Patient safety in the pediatric emergency care setting. *Pediatrics* 120:1367–1375, 2007.

7. Fernandez C.V., Gills-Ring J.: Strategies for the prevention of medical error in pediatrics. *J Pediatr* 143:155–162, 2003.

8. France D.J., Levin S., Hemphill R., et al.: Emergency physicians' behaviors and workload in the presence of an electronic whiteboard. *Int J Med Inform* 74:827–837, 2005.

9. Woloshynowych M., Davis R., Brown R., et al.: Communication patterns in a UK emergency department. *Ann Emerg Med* 50:407–413, 2007.

10. Spenser R., Coiera E., Logan P.: Variation in communication loads on clinical staff in the emergency department. *Annals of Emergency Medicine* 44(3):268–73, 2004.

11. American Academy of Pediatrics Committee on Emergency Medicine, American College of Emergency Physicians Pediatric Committee: Care of Children in the Emergency Department: Guidelines for Preparedness. *Pediatrics* 107(4)777–781, 2001.

12. Shaw K.N., Lavelle J., Crescenzo K., et al.: Creating unit-based patient safety walk-rounds in a pediatric emergency department. *Clinical Pediatric Emergency Medicine* 7(4)231, 2006.

13. Williams M.V., Parker R.M., Baker D.W., et al.: Inadequate functional health literacy among patients at two public hospitals. *JAMA* 274:1677–1682, 1995.

14. Taveras E.M., Flores G.: Why culture and language matter: The clinical consequences of providing culturally and linguistically appropriate services to children in the emergency department. Clinical Pediatric Emergency Medicine 5(2):76–84, 2004.

15. Wiener, E.S., Rivera, M.I.: Bridging language barriers: how to work with an interpreter. *Clinical Pediatric Emergency Medicine* 5(2):93–102, 2004.

16. Jacobs E.A., Chen A.H., Karliner L., et al.: Legal and regulatory obligations to provide culturally and linguistically appropriate emergency department services. *Clinical Pediatric Emergency Medicine* 5(2):85–92, 2004.

17. Sexton J.B., Thomas E.J., et al.: Error, stress and teamwork in medicine and aviation. *BMJ* 320:745–749, 2000.

18. Selbst S.M., Levine S., et al.: Preventing medical errors in pediatric emergency medicine. *Pediatr Emerg Care* 20(10):702–708, 2004.

19. Federwisch A.: Bedside Shift Report Ensures Quality Handoff. Nurse.com Home Page, November 20, 2007, http://include.nurse.com/apps/pbcs.dll/article?AID=/20071120/MS02/311200030 (accessed Nov. 20, 2007).

20. Patterson E.S., Roth E.M., Woods D.D., et al.: Handoff strategies in settings with high consequences for failure: lessons for health care operations. *International Journal for Quality in Health Care* 16(2):125–32, 2004.

21. Apker J., Mallak L.A., Gibson S.C.: Communicating in the "gray zone": Perceptions about emergency physician hospitalist handoffs and patient safety. *Acad Emerg Med* 14:884–894, 2007.

22. Shendell-Falik N., Feinson M., Mohr B.J.: Enhancing patient safety: Improving the patient handoff process through appreciative inquiry. *J Nurs Adm* 37:95–104, 2007.

23. Laxmisan A., Hakimzada F., Sayan O.R., et al.: The multitasking clinician: decision-making and cognitive demand during and after team handoffs in emergency care. *Int J Med Inform* 76:801–811, 2007.

24. Viccellio P. and ACEP task force report on Boarding. Emergency Department Crowding: High-Impact Solutions. www.ACEP.org (accessed Sep. 1, 2008).

25. Hospital Survey on Patient Safety Culture: 2007 Comparative Database Report http://www.ahrq.gov/qual/hospsurveydb/hospsurveydb2.pdf (accessed Feb. 24, 2008).

26. Strategies to improve hand-off communication: Implementing a process to resolve questions. *Joint Commission Perspectives on Patient Safety* 5(7):11, July 2005.

27. The Joint Commission: *Improving Hand-off Communication.* Oakbrook Terrace, IL: Joint Commission Resources, pp. 15–16, 2007.

28. Gawande A.: The checklist: If something so simple can transform intensive care, what else can it do? *The New Yorker,* Dec. 10, 2007. http://www.newyorker.com/reporting/2007/12/10/071210fa_fact_gawande (accessed Jul. 21, 2009).

29. Committee on Pediatric Emergency Medicine, American Academy of Pediatrics. Emergency preparedness for children with special health care needs. *Pediatrics* 104:e53, 1999.

30. Shapiro J.S., Kannry J., Lipton M., et al.: Approaches to patient health information exchange and their impact on emergency medicine. *Ann Emerg Med* 48:426–432, 2006.

31. The Success of Just-in-Time Emergency Department Access to Patient Medication Information History. Available online at http://www.surescript.com/downloads/regenstrief_initiate_rxhub .pdf (accessed Jul. 21, 2009).

32. Albanese S.A.: From the cockpit to the OR. American Academy of Orthopaedic Surgeons Home Page, www.aaos.org/news/ bulletin/sep07/managing6.asp (accessed Nov. 28, 2007).

33. Gallagher T.H., Waterman A.D., Ebers A.G., et al.: Patients' and physicians' attitudes regarding the disclosure of medical errors. *JAMA* 289:1001–1007, 2003.

34. Wu A.W., Folkman S., McPhee S.J., et al.: Do house officers learn from their mistakes? *JAMA* 265(16):2089–2094, Apr. 24, 1991. UI: 2013929.

35. O'Neill K.A.: Kids speak: Effective communication with the school-aged/adolescent patient. *Pediatr Emerg Care* 18(2):137–138, 2002.

36. Levinson W.: Doctor-patient communication and medical malpractice for pediatricians. *Pediatr Ann* 26(3):186–193, 1997.

37. American Academy of Pediatrics, Committee on Pediatric Emergency Medicine, American College of Emergency Physicians Pediatric Emergency Medicine Committee. Patient- and family-centered care and the role of the emergency physician providing care to a child in the emergency department. *Pediatrics;* 118(5): 2242–2244 (doi:10.1542/peds.2006–2588), 2006.

CHAPTER 3

Promoting a Patient and Family-Centered Environment of Care® in the ED

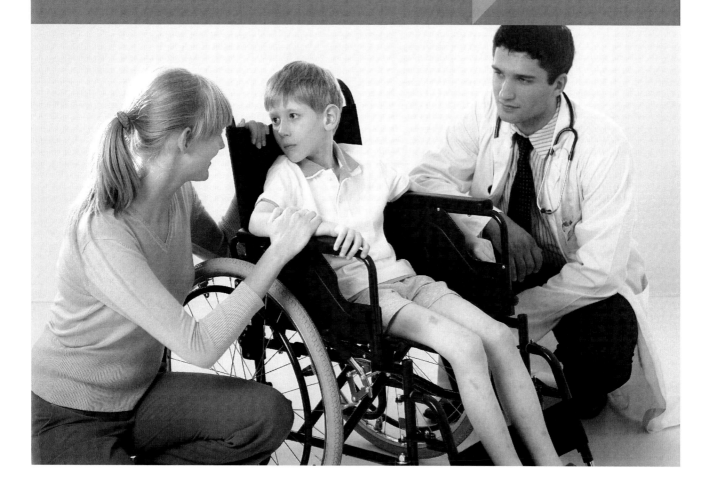

Contributing Editor: Francine Westergaard, R.N., M.S.N., M.B.A., *consultant for Joint Commission International and Joint Commission Resources*

When they arrive in the emergency department (ED), children and their parents are typically filled with anxiety, fear, and confusion. Stress levels may be increased as the patient and his or her family may have no previous experience with the ED or relationship with the health care providers. In some situations, children may not be accompanied by a parent or guardian if they are transferred by ambulance, adding to their stress. In a fast-paced environment that is often filled with distractions and interruptions, tension and trauma, pediatric patients and their families require attention to their comfort as well as medical care. This chapter explores strategies and techniques ED staff can employ to effectively manage the ED environment and deliver patient- and family-centered care (PFCC), and in doing so, leverage PFCC as a strategy to improve pediatric care quality and patient safety.

Adopting Family-Centered Care in the ED

Patient- and family-centered care acknowledges the significance of the role of the family in the care of a patient and promotes a collaborative approach to patient well-being between the patient, family, and health care professionals. PFCC embraces the following concepts[1]:

- Care is provided for a person, not just a condition.

- The patient is best understood in the context of his or her family, culture, values, and goals.

- Honoring the context will result in better health care quality, safety, and patient satisfaction.

- To optimize a child's care, ED providers, parents, and the child are all on the same team.

ED staff are frequently challenged with circumstances unique to emergency medicine. As discussed in Chapter 1, most EDs face conditions of overcrowding that result in a chaotic environment with frequent workflow interruptions. Serving a large volume of patients on an unscheduled and somewhat unpredictable basis creates a variety of challenges that range from limited staffing and space to limited available time for gaining sufficient patient information.[2] These and other factors clearly contribute to an increased risk of medical error in the ED. These same factors challenge the provision of PFCC.

Although health care staff in other settings (such as an operating room, clinic, diagnostic suite, or outpatient surgical center) manage one patient at a time, emergency care professionals are often responsible for the simultaneous management of multiple patients with a variety of problems and varying levels of acuity.[2] It perhaps goes without saying that ED personnel often work under a great deal of stress. Children are, of course, at particular risk under these circumstances because of their physical and developmental vulnerabilities and their inability to accurately describe their symptoms and past medical history. These factors unique to children also appear to increase risk for medical error.

Children often receive care from emergency care providers who may not be accustomed to treating pediatric patients. Many community EDs do not have designated pediatric providers or examination facilities. Nearly 90% of children receive their emergency care in a non-children's hospital setting.[3] Half of these EDs care for fewer than 10 children per day. As critically ill or injured children represent only a small percentage (generally less than 10%) of all pediatric ED visits, ED providers in these settings may not have an opportunity to maintain their clinical skills in the assessment and treatment of severely ill children.[3]

In its 2006 publication, *Emergency Care for Children: Growing Pains,* the Institute of Medicine identified PFCC as a strategy to improve pediatric care quality and patient safety in the ED. The report offers a strong endorsement, noting that the failure to incorporate PFCC and culturally effective care into ED practice "can result in multiple adverse consequences, including difficulties with informed consent, miscommunication, inadequate understanding of diagnoses and treatment by families, dissatisfaction with care, preventable morbidity and mortality, unnecessary child abuse evaluations, lower quality care, clinician bias, and ethnic disparities in prescriptions, analgesia, test ordering, and diagnostic evaluation."[4]

In an effort to offset some of the common challenges associated with the delivery of pediatric patient care in the ED, many organizations have adopted a family-centered approach to ED care. As discussed in Chapter 2, engaging and involving pediatric patients and their families in the course of care helps clinicians build trust with patients, which can aid the process of information-gathering, communication, and treatment. In a family-centered setting that succeeds in reducing the anxiety of pediatric patients and their families, staff expand their control over the ED environment of care and, therefore, are able to function more efficiently. For example, less time spent policing visitors allows more time for patient contact and improves job satisfaction.[5]

In addition to benefits offered to patients and families, PFCC also appears to be associated with a number of benefits for health care providers, including: improved clinical-decision making; greater satisfaction with workplace environment; improved understanding of social, ethnic, and cultural diversity; improved awareness of the needs of children with special health care needs; and reductions in medical error and liability risk. Improved clinical decision-making may serve to reduce error, or may help to improve clinical efficiency, assisting with ED throughput. Improved staff satisfaction may serve to reduce burnout and turnover rates. Lower liability risk may be secondary to more informed and less error-prone clinical decisions, or perhaps a more careful or deliberate process with family present. It may also be the result of greater trust and family satisfaction with ED care providers.[6]

ED leaders who encourage the addition of patient and family member representatives to department committees responsible for the development and implementation of PFCC policies and procedures will build valuable relationships. These PFCC committees will provide insight into policy development for visitation, family presence during procedures, comfort care, language translation, cultural competency, and patient and family satisfaction. These committees bring great value to health care facilities as they plan for PFCC at all levels from daily operations to facility design.[7] Parents and family members can provide valuable insight into planning for their presence during health care procedures, including resuscitation, involvement in post procedure care of the child, knowledge transfer during the discharge process, pediatric quality initiatives, and patient satisfaction. This is particularly significant for families with children with special health care needs. When a child with special health care needs presents to the ED, they will clearly benefit when their families are able to effectively partner with health care providers.

The Institute for Family Centered Care has identified the following as the core principles of family-centered care[8]:

• Treating patients and families with dignity and respect

• Communication of unbiased information

• Patient and family participation in experiences that enhance control and independence and build on their strengths

• Collaboration in the delivery of care, policy and program development, and professional education

Embracing a family-centered approach to care "moves the focus of health care professionals from family deficits to strengths, control to collaboration, expert model to partnerships, information gate-keeping to information sharing, negative support to positive support, rigidity to flexibility, and patient/family dependence to empowerment."[9] PFCC relies on collaboration between patients, their families, and health care professionals, and acknowledges that a patient's family is a constant in the patient's life and an essential part of the care process. Because each family is unique due to many factors, including ethnic, racial, spiritual, social, economic, educational, and geographic diversities, a family's methods of coping are supported by staff and the range of their strengths, concerns, emotions, and aspirations are recognized.[1,9]

The checklist in Sidebar 3-1, page 44, provides steps for implementing family-centered care into a department or organization.

Supporting Family Presence During All Aspects of Care

A fundamental component of PFCC for children in the ED is maintaining the presence of parents and other key family members during all aspects of care. Considerations for the resources and processes to support family presence should begin with the arrival of the patient to the ED. A parent that transports their child to the ED should not be forced to leave their child to park a car. Triage processes should allow the presence of parents or guardians, as they will be vital sources of information in determining illness acuity. Patient registration should never require the separation of a parent from their child. ED examinations rooms should likewise accommodate family members.

There is a growing awareness of the many benefits afforded by PFCC practices to patients, family, and staff.[10,11] One evolving area in PFCC is a practice that promotes the presence of family members during invasive procedures and resuscitation. There are a growing number of published studies on ED family presence in peer-reviewed journals which indicate that 60% to 80% of families believe they want to be present during care. Surveys of ED health care providers have found them somewhat less supportive of family presence, with nurses being generally more supportive than physicians, and senior physicians more supportive than trainees.[11]

Inexperienced staff may be reluctant to have family members present in these settings fearing that this might serve to reduce their efficacy during a technical procedure. Another frequently offered concern is that family presence might result in a delay or disruption of care. Interestingly, published reports of family presence trials in EDs have not demonstrated this to be a significant concern.[6,10,11] Getting beyond this fear might be a vital step, as the literature indicates that healthcare providers who initially oppose family presence commonly become fierce advocates after trying it.

Support for family presence during emergency care and resuscitation can now be found in policy statements of key professional organizations, including the American Heart Association (AHA), American Academy of Pediatrics, American College of Emergency Physicians and Emergency Nurses Association. PFCC can also be found in published guidelines for emergency and resuscitative care, including

| Sidebar 3-1 | **Checklist for Implementing Family-Centered Care** |

The following checklist may be used to evaluate the needs of families and prepare for implementation of a family-centered care model.

☐ **Evaluate the needs of families served by the ED.**

Surveys, conversations with families, focus groups, and/or family advisory committees are strategies to gather this information.

☐ **Develop a department mission, vision, and philosophy of care that includes PFCC principles.**

Articulating a family-centered care, mission, vision, and philosophy for the ED provides structure to help direct change and establishes PFCC as a core value. Creating an interdisciplinary group to formulate these statements is an excellent opportunity to involve ED staff, administrators, physicians, and external departments who provide services to ED families (e.g., social work, pediatricians and pediatric subspecialists, radiology, respiratory care, phlebotomy, pharmacy, pastoral care, child life, volunteer services, and ancillary departments).

☐ **Evaluate department policies and procedures for congruency with PFCC principles.**

Organizations should routinely evaluate how they approach PFCC challenges, including overcrowding; patient flow; security and identification of family members; family presence during procedures, including resuscitation; interpretation services; routine comfort care; coordination of communication and care with the child's medical home; discharge planning and instructions; the physical environment of the ED.[1]

☐ **Educate ED staff on family needs, communication, health literacy, cultural competency, and the family perspective.**

Ongoing staff education regarding family issues and family-centered care can be provided through a variety of formats, including in-service education, bulletin board postings, department-based newsletters, journal clubs, and feedback from patient surveys. Modeling the expected behaviors is essential to the integration of the approach. Use the expertise of staff committed to the process within the hospital or community to assist with education and program development. This can be accomplished through the use of pediatric patient champions in the ED.[2]

☐ **Engage family members to assist with the education of staff on cultural competency and the family perspective.**

☐ **Develop staff competencies related to PFCC.**

☐ **Provide an environment that is child and family friendly, including furnishings, fixtures, and the availability of age-appropriate toys and play activities.[3]**

A welcoming and comfortable environment is important to the patient and family. A physical environment that can accommodate the entire family including siblings and extended family members should be strived for. Also, when possible, providing an environment for children and their families free of distressing sights and sounds often found in the ED will help ease anxiety and fear for children and their families.

References

1. O'Malley P., Brown K., Krug S., and the American Academy of Pediatrics Committee on Pediatric Emergency Medicine: Patient and family centered care of children in the emergency department. *Pediatrics* 122(3):e511–e521, 2008.
2. Nadzam D., Westergaard F.: Pediatric patient safety in the emergency department: Identifying risks and preparing to care for child and family. *J Nurs Care Qual* 23(3):189–194, 2008.
3. Gausche-Hill M., Schmitz C., Lewis R.J.: Pediatric preparedness of United States emergency departments: a 2003 survey. *Pediatrics* 120:1229–1237, 2007.

Adapted from Assessment of Family-Centered Care in the Emergency Department. Emergency Nurses Association, Health Resources and Services Administration, Emergency Medical Services for Children, http://www.ena.org.

the AHA cardiopulmonary resuscitation guidelines, Pediatric Advanced Life Support, Advanced Pediatric Life Support, and the Emergency Nursing Pediatric Course and Trauma Nursing Core Course.

Guzzetta and colleagues offer guidance to EDs that wish to extend their PFCC practices to more challenging clinical scenarios, including resuscitation.[11] They advocate the development of an ED policy on family presence, which entails the discussion of this practice within all disciplines. This practice recognizes the potential benefits afforded to children and their family members, but also allows any involved care team member to veto family presence if they feel compromised. This best practice also includes some screening and preparation of family (whenever possible) and enlists the support of a staff member whose primary role is to support the family members during the event.

Initiating Child Life Programs

In working to provide children with a safe environment of care in the ED, organizations have also integrated Child Life specialists into their ED services. According to the American Academy of Pediatrics, "The Child Life specialist focuses on the strengths and sense of well-being of children while promoting their optimal development and minimizing the adverse effects of children's experiences in health care or other potentially stressful settings."[12]

Child Life specialists use play and psychological preparation as their primary interventions during stressful and sometimes overwhelming moments for pediatric patients. By doing so, they help relieve stress and facilitate coping and adjustment. Play and age-appropriate communication may be used to support the following[12]:

- Promotion of optimal child development
- Presentation of clear and unbiased information
- Identification and rehearsing of useful coping strategies for medical events or procedures
- Helping patients and families work through feelings about past or impending experiences
- Establishment of therapeutic relationships with children and parents to support family involvement in each child's care, with continuity across the care continuum
- Implementation of distraction techniques during painful procedures and to enhance cooperation with exams and procedures

Child Life can also work with siblings to help them prepare for what they will see when visiting their sibling.

The Child Life Council, a national organization of Child Life specialists that determines the profession's certification criteria, recommends that child life services should be considered an essential component of quality pediatric health care and integral to family-centered care and best-practice models of health care delivery for children. Child life services should be performed in collaboration with and give support to the child's medical home.[12]

The following case study chronicles the role of a Child Life specialist at American Family Children's Hospital in Madison, Wisconsin, which is part of the health system for the University of Wisconsin (UW).

In enhancing the effectiveness of Child Life initiatives, organizations should consider positioning a Child Life specialist as a partner along with a nurse-physician team that guides the process of pediatric care in the ED. The Child Life specialist can help design a setting in which nurses and physicians can more effectively care for children and families. Going beyond creature comforts such as a waiting area decorated and stocked with child-sized furnishings, Child Life specialists can also provide valued assistance with painful or frightening procedures and with patient care education.

In fact, through its Child Life program, UW's American Family Children's Hospital offers constructive distraction for the siblings of pediatric patients. Club Sibs is a weekly program that brings together the brothers and sisters ages 6 to 12 years of hospitalized children to talk about the hospital and engage in fun projects, including art therapy and activities such as those featured in Sidebar 3-2, page 47.

Child Life experts can provide assistance to ED leaders in determining what toys or play materials (e.g., coloring books, picture books, board games) would be best to meet the needs of pediatric patients and their siblings. The presence of a television with child appropriate videos or programming in the ED exam room may be greatly appreciated by children and their families. In initiating a kinder and gentler approach to care, Child Life specialists can help ED staff provide effective and family-centered pediatric emergency care thereby enhancing patient and family satisfaction.[13]

Providing Comfort for Children in Distress

One of the realities of pediatric emergency care is the many interventions that can result in pain or anxiety. Even for those children who do not require needlesticks or other painful diagnostic procedures, the simple presence of ED staff may promote great distress. As already discussed, advocating for family presence and promoting a child friendly environment may help. Of course, as children of different ages have different developmental capabilities and coping mechanisms, there is no single intervention that works for all children. An innovative intervention developed by Cathy Shanahan, R.N., the director of

Case Study 3-1

Child Life Services in the Emergency Department

Confused. Anxious. Scared. When a child arrives to the ED at the University of Wisconsin (UW) Hospital, any or all of the above words may be used to describe his or her frame of mind. Thrust into an unfamiliar environment, one that often consists of rapid movement and strange voices and sounds, the child's fear may lead to behavior changes, such as crying, fussing, or even tantrums, making emergency treatment a difficult task for ED staff. This is why the UW's children's hospital hired their Child Life specialist, Lisa Peck.

Peck joined the children's hospital as a Child Life specialist in a position created specifically to address the needs of children in the ED. Her role is to use her extensive training to make the child's and family's time in the ED as stress- and worry-free as possible.

"We all know that the environment in the emergency department isn't very child-friendly," Peck says. "My job is to try to lower anxiety levels of the patient and parents." She achieves this in a number of ways. When children are brought to the ED, Peck immediately assesses the situation and decides upon a specific course of action. If the ED physicians determine that the patient needs to undergo a procedure, such as an X-ray or computed tomography scan, she may explain to the child what the procedure entails. When children can comprehend their surroundings, their level of fear often decreases, and their resistance subsides.

"I talk to them about what they're going to see and what their job is," Peck says. "The more children understand what is going to happen, the better they do with the procedure."

Diversion also plays a substantial role in helping to reroute the child's attention away from treatment interventions that might be painful. Peck shows movies or offers the patient a hand-held game system with which he or she can use to occupy their fingers and minds.

For children with broken bones, she produces a doll with a removable cast, and demonstrates where the cast will go and what it will look like while making clear the reasons for its necessity. She is also planning on developing a series of preparatory books that she can use in the ED to enlighten patients about certain surgical procedures they may need to endure.

Child Life specialists provide developmentally appropriate information to assist children in understanding and coping with the hospital environment. Peck graduated from the University of Iowa with a degree in therapeutic recreation but had to complete a 480-hour internship at the school to be eligible for her current position. The internship is one of the qualifications set forth by the Child Life Council, a national organization of Child Life specialists that determines the profession's certification criteria. In addition to the internship, Child Life specialists must hold a bachelor's degree and have taken a minimum of 10 courses in Child Life, child development, child and family studies or closely related areas. To maintain certification, specialists must pass the Child Life Professional Certification Examination at least once every 10 years.

Mary Kaminski, the Child Life Services manager who hired Peck, believes her integration of the children's hospital's concept of care in the UW ED will pay dividends in the arena of patient satisfaction.

"I think we offer something very special for children," Kaminski says. :The psychosocial needs that children have when they go through a fearful, stressful event will certainly be addressed, and interventions will be delivered so children can cope with the setting and the experience, and leave with a positive, healthy mindset."

Peck agrees, saying, "I think Child Life is definitely going to grow and succeed. Every emergency department is striving to improve itself and make their patients happier. I think Child Life will help do that."

Reprinted with permission from American Family Children's Hospital, Madison, Wisconsin.

emergency services at Children's Memorial Hospital, in partnership with the hospital's Child Life services, is the Comfort Cart.

"The experience of illness is not a normal part of childhood and although we cannot eliminate all pain and anxiety associated with medical treatment our commitment to our families is to minimize the unpleasant experience to the best of our ability," says Shanahan. "We partner with patients and families to develop an individualized and multidimensional approach to pain management that allows for choice and comfort. It is our expectation that caregivers throughout our hospital are responsive and sensitive to the needs of patients and families."

Activities for the Siblings of Pediatric Patients

"I'm bored ..."
Sometimes it's hard for children and siblings to think of things to do in the hospital while waiting for the completion of treatment or waiting for a brother or sister to be released. Here are some ideas to suggest to siblings who have accompanied the patient in the ED examination room, or for those in the waiting room.

Things to do in the hospital

- Read a book
- Make a craft for yourself or for your brother/sister
- Paint, color, or draw a picture
- Play a board game
- Play a card game
- Finish your homework
- Play on the computer
- Make a journal of your trip to the hospital
- Write a letter
- Sing to your brother/sister
- Put together a puzzle
- Listen to music
- Give your mom and/or dad a break and stay with your brother/sister
- Play a video game
- Watch TV or a movie

Adapted from Child Life Services in the Emergency Department. UW Health Home Page, http://www.uwhealth.org/page.asp?contentid=11660 (accessed Nov. 16, 2007). Reprinted with permission from American Family Children's Hospital, Madison, Wisconsin.

Contents of Comfort Cart at Children's Memorial Hospital

Comfort Items for Babies and Toddlers
Rattles
Books on animals
Rain stick
Magnetic doodle pad

Comfort Items for Visual Distraction
Bubble maker
Handheld electronic games
Handheld photo viewer and slides
Glitter wand
Squeeze balls

Comfort Items to Use and Give Away
Pinwheels
Assorted stickers

Music and Books for Various Ages
CD Player with CDs, including nature sounds, classical music, and children's songs
Assorted books

Administrative Items
Comfort cards that provide comfort tips and strategies
Supply ordering information
Comfort protocols
Age-specific algorithms for using comfort techniques
Resource list of Child Life specialists

Adapted from "Using and Maintaining the Comfort Carts." Children's Memorial Hospital, Chicago. Printed with permission.

"The ultimate outcome of this project is to have a 'pain-free' children's hospital with a goal toward satisfying the needs of families and children. The purpose of the carts is to create a more consistent approach to non-sedated, invasive procedures that cause pain, fear and anxiety for our patients and their families. We expect this approach will promote an atmosphere that will reduce the fear and anxiety associated with potentially painful procedures."

The Comfort Carts are stocked with a variety of items that help to soothe distressed children (and their families), including toys, books, audio and video devices, handheld games, various gadgets, and other fun items (such as a bubble maker and spinning wheels) that help to provide distraction or comfort for children of all ages. The Comfort Cart intervention was begun in the ED but has since been implemented hospital-wide. Sidebar 3-3, above, lists the contents of a Comfort Cart at Children's Memorial Hospital.

The Collaborative Health Care Team

The pediatric health care team is an expansive and inclusive one. Emergency care coordination typically includes team members from multiple disciplines, including medicine, nursing, pharmacy, social service, chaplains, case managers, respiratory care, diagnostics, and the patient and family. Coordination of care beyond the ED encounter requires the inclusion of the patient's medical home and any subspecialists involved in the child's care.[14] Valuable information about the patient, and particularly for medically complex children, can be obtained from these sources. Input from the child's medical home can help determine appropriate treatment and disposition.

Pharmacists can be valuable team members during the medication reconciliation process and in support of the medication delivery process while an ill child is in the ED. Respiratory care practitioners can likewise bring great value in the emergency care of the pediatric patient because many children present with acute respiratory care needs. Social workers and case managers can be instrumental in facilitating the discharge planning of a child particularly those with complex, special health care needs that are supplemented with medical technology in the home environment. Chaplains can provide crucial support to families in need during visits to the ED. A well-coordinated multidisciplinary ED care team that is committed to providing PFCC should serve to improve pediatric clinical outcomes, promote ED staff and family satisfaction, and optimize patient safety.

Improving Pediatric Safety in the ED

In pursuit of strategies to enhance the environment of care in the ED, organizations have to examine all of the practices and processes that support the treatment provided—from whether inpatient nurses with pediatric experience come to assist staff with care if a child is in the ED for an extended period of time or is undergoing a difficult procedure, to the ways in which clinical documentation is carried out in the ED. As part of this evaluation, the ED facility and its equipment deserve consideration for how they support PFCC and the unique hazards they may pose for pediatric patients and family members. Sidebar 3-4, page 50, discusses additional suggestions for keeping children safe in the ED.

Improving Flow by Standardizing and Sustaining ED Processes

Although it may seem somewhat insignificant, standardized processes and paperwork that are necessary to provide safe care can also impact the flow in the ED. Just as these key processes should not be skipped by front-line staff in efforts to save time, ED leadership should not ignore these processes or systems as they consider patient safety improvement. Too often, ED staff are forced to share a limited number of sometimes unreliable computers and must wait for their turn to access them for such tasks as charting and obtaining patient information. Limited access to electronic patient information can result in medical error and delays in care. Other ED operation considerations, including making sure that staff don't have to travel far from their patients to access supplies, may go a long way in reducing staff fatigue and even the time patients and families spend in the waiting room. As an example, isolation carts, pediatric vascular access carts, or procedure carts should be accessible to staff and there should be enough carts to meet patient demand. The use of specialized carts (versus specialized treatment areas) may also help to limit the need to move patients from one room to another. This may also promote PFCC and patient satisfaction.

Taking Measures to Prevent Patient Abduction and Elopement

Organizations and their personnel also have to consider the potential of patient abduction and elopement in all clinical areas, including the ED. The Joint Commission highlighted its concern on this issue in December 2004 by approving new language that added the abduction of any individual receiving care, treatment, or services to the list of its reviewable sentinel events. This change broadened a previous requirement, infant abduction, and this continues to apply to all healthcare organizations, including acute care hospitals, psychiatric hospitals, hospice facilities, subacute care facilities, nursing homes, clinics, counseling centers, and other outpatient settings. Organizations must consider processes that enhance the security for pediatric patients in the ED.[14] This can be accomplished through the establishment of a process to identify family members separate from other visitors. In addition, health care providers must be cognizant of how to work effectively with families when the family disagrees with the proposed treatment plan. This includes providing a clear and unbiased understanding of benefits and risks, including potential complications. Parents (and when developmentally appropriate, patients) must be well informed and should be encouraged to remain involved in the care process. These efforts may help to reduce the likelihood that a family might elect to leave the ED without completion of necessary medical treatment.

Case Study 3-2

Tabletop Abduction Drill

As Washington State's only psychiatric hospital for children, Child Study and Treatment Center in Lakewood, Washington, is a long-term inpatient facility for children ages 5 to 17. The Center houses 47 inpatient beds in three cottages that are locked 24 hours a day. In the behavioral health unit, day treatment is provided to 17 children, who receive psychiatric services and attend school on campus. The Center's length of stay averages between 6 and 9 months, and the hospital is home to the state's most psychiatrically impaired young patients.

Although the facility is locked, many children take part in activities both on and off campus, which means multiple opportunities for abduction. The Center's safety chair is Erik Logan, who says, "Our kids have a lot of legal custody issues, but so far there have been no abductions. Nevertheless, we want to stay on top of the issue."

An abduction-prevention procedure was first put in place more than six years ago. Shortly after that, the Center's staff conducted a mock drill designed to test their preparedness.

Unfortunately, it was not as successful as they had hoped. "It proved too stressful for the patients," Logan recalls. "We realized it would be better if we did the drill on paper so we don't make things worse for the kids."

Recently, the Center's staff updated the procedure and changed it from a mock drill into a tabletop drill. In that procedure, a staff member from each cottage was given a written scenario about a 15-year-old girl involved in a custody battle between her parents. The girl was on her way to a dental appointment with staff when a man grabbed her by the wrist and ran with her to a waiting car that then sped off.

Designated staff members had to notify law enforcement and give them the make, model, and license number of the vehicle, a description of the abductor, and a description of the patient, along with her medical background and her status at the Center. Finally,

they had to complete the paperwork, including an incident report and an unauthorized leave form.

Holly Galbreath, Ph.D., is the program director for one of the Center's three cottages. "One reason the tabletop drill was so successful is that we designed it to resemble the drills already in use for runaways, which are far more common than abductions," she says. "That was really helpful to the staff, and we plan to repeat the drill each year." Galbreath credits Logan with much of the design work. She points out that there are difficulties inherent in preparing for an event such as an abduction, which everyone hopes will never happen. Says Galbreath, "A drill will probably be a lot easier for facilities if they make it similar to something that's more common so there's less for the staff to learn."

Following the Joint Commission standards, hospitals are required to identify and manage their security risks, including implementing security procedures that address handling of an infant or pediatric abduction, as applicable. According to Jerry Gervais, C.H.S.P., C.H.F.M., Associate Director, Standards Interpretation Group, Joint Commission, the following phrase as applicable is key: "Hospitals and other health care facilities will take different approaches to meet their security needs, depending on the location they serve. Urban, suburban, and rural areas may all face different concerns."

As an example, Gervais cites hospitals and health care facilities in areas where visitors sometimes come in carrying weapons. "When the Joint Commission arrives for a survey, we don't necessarily understand the security concerns of that individual hospital. That's why we ask organizations to do an assessment of their needs before establishing a policy and a plan to prevent abduction."

With care, repeated drills, ongoing training, and unflagging watchfulness, there is a reasonable expectation that health care organizations will be able to prevent abduction and assure the safety of infants, pediatric patients, and adolescents.

Source: Joint Commission Resources: Keeping young patients safe: Preventing abduction of pediatric and adolescent patients. *Environment of Care News* 8:8, Nov. 2005.

In recent years the issue of child abduction has also been magnified by the enactment of Megan's Law and the nationwide use of Amber Alerts. Both of these prevention mechanisms are named in memory of abducted and

murdered children and provide the public with information on the whereabouts of sex offenders so that local communities can protect their children.

Sidebar 3-4	What EDs Can Do to Keep Children Safe

Child-Proofing the ED

During a family crisis, such as the acute illness or injury of a child, the whole family may accompany the patient to the hospital for treatment. These family members often include other children of various ages, from infants to school-age children. Most EDs contain equipment and supplies that may be hazardous for child visitors, particularly toddlers and pre-school-aged children. For PFCC to be plausible the environment must be safe for family members, including children. "If you want to see an ED from a child's perspective, get down on your hands and knees," suggests Dr. Tony Woodward, Chief of Emergency Medicine at Seattle Children's Hospital. "The floors and walls can be a minefield for children." Among the child hazards he cites are:

- Suction canisters

- Dirty laundry

- Electrical outlets into which a child can insert a finger or a metal object

- Supply drawers or sharps containers that can be pried open by tiny hands

- Stray pills and other hazards that fall to the floor

- Medical tools and equipment

- Spilled blood and other body fluids

- Unsecure, hazardous cleaning agents

- Low waste cans containing infectious waste

Francine Westergaard R.N., M.S.N., consultant for Joint Commission International and Joint Commission Resources, suggests, "Be sure to position supply drawers and sharps containers where children can't reach them—perhaps affixed to the wall, well above a child's reach." Dr. Richard Molteni, former medical director, Seattle Children's Hospital, adds he's amazed by how often items in an ED are located at a height that may be appropriate for an adult but from where children may still be able to reach a cord and pull down items on top of themselves. He also suggests eliminating any sharp edges that a child can encounter and avoiding carpeted flooring because carpet can soak up spills and chemical residues from cleaning agents that could be infectious or harmful for infants still in the crawling stage. In addition, he says, "most of the beds used in many EDs are adult size, and even with the side rails up, children can climb out and fall."

Create a Child-Friendly Environment

Molteni also suggests that EDs can help promote patient comfort by creating a soothing environment that will distract children from their fear, distress, and pain. He suggests adding pictures on the ceilings, bright colors on the walls, and a television in exam rooms offering child-appropriate programming. Organizations should consider the addition of services that will allow pediatric programming. This programming should be multilingual to meet the needs of the population served. "It's really helpful for hospitals to create a patient room in which children can be cared for and even entertained safely."

Source: Joint Commission Resources: Pediatric safety in emergencies: what health care organizations can do to keep children safe. *Environment of Care News* 11:1–3, Feb. 2008.

References

1. Mace S., Brown K., and the American Academy of Pediatrics, Committee on Pediatric Emergency Medicine, American College of Emergency Physicians and Pediatric Emergency Medicine Committee: Patient and family-centered care and the role of the emergency physician providing care to a child in the emergency department. *Pediatrics* 115(5):2242–2244, 2006.

2. Committee on the Future of Emergency Care in the United States Health System: *Emergency care for children: growing pains.* Washington, D.C.: National Academies Press, 2007. Available at: http://books.nap.edu/openbook.php?record_id=11655&page=R1.

3. Gausche-Hill M., Schmitz C., Lewis R.J.: Pediatric preparedness of United States emergency departments: a 2003 survey. *Pediatrics* 120:1229–1237, 2007.

4. Institute of Medicine: *Emergency care for children: Growing pains.* Washington, D.C.: National Academies Press, 2006.

5. Piskosz Z.: One pediatric emergency department's approach to family-centered-care. *J Emerg Nurs* 33(2):169–170, 2007.

6. Krug S.E.: Family-centered care and patient safety of children in the emergency department. American Academy of Pediatrics Safer Healthcare for Kids Webinar, June 21, 2007. Available at: www.aap.org.

7. Eichner J., Johnson B., American Academy of Pediatrics, Committee on Hospital Care: Family-centered care and the pediatrician's role. *Pediatrics* 1112(3), 691–696, 2003.

8. Institute for Family Centered Care: Core principles of family-centered health care. *Adv Fam Centered Care* 4:2–4, 1998.

9. Assessment of Family-Centered Care in the Emergency Department. Emergency Nurses Association, Health Resources and Services Administration, Emergency Medical Services for Children. Available at: http://www.ena.org/pdf/Guidelines.PDF (accessed Dec. 3, 2007).

10. Sacchetti A., Guzzetta C., Harris R.: Family presence during resuscitation attempts and invasive procedures: is there science behind the emotion. *Clin Pediatr Emerg Med* 4(4): 292–301, 2003.

11. Guzzetta C.E., Clark A.P., Wright J.L.: Family presence in emergency medical services for children. *Clin Pediatr Emerg Med* 7(1):15–24, 2006.

12. Child Life Council and American Academy of Pediatrics Committee on Hospital Care: Child life services. *Pediatrics* 118(4):1757–1763, 2006.

13. Coleman P.: Management of the pediatric patient in the adult emergency department. The Virginia Henderson International Nursing Library Home Page, 2003. Available at: http://www.nursinglibrary.org/Portal/main.aspx?pageid=4024&pid=10566 (accessed Nov. 17, 2007).

14. O'Malley P., Brown K., Krug S., American Academy of Pediatrics Committee on Pediatric Emergency Medicine: Patient and family centered care of children in the emergency department. *Pediatrics* 122(3):e511–e521, 2008.

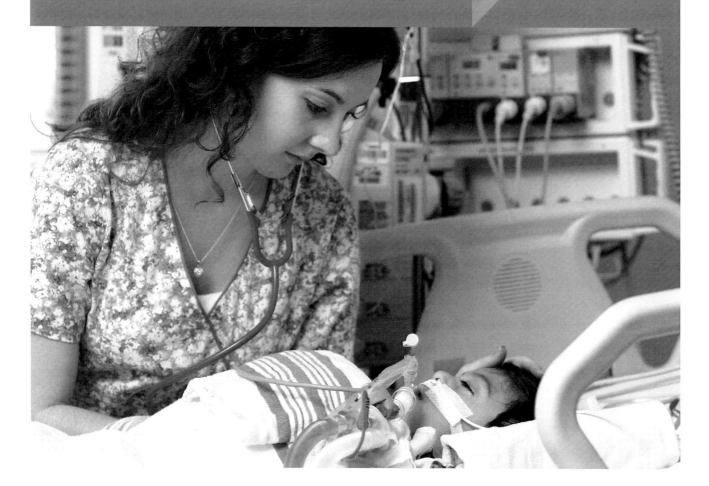

CHAPTER 4

Medication Safety for Pediatric Patients in the Emergency Department

Authored by Jeannell Mansur, R.Ph., Pharm.D., F.A.S.H.P., *practice leader, medication safety, Joint Commission Resources*

Recent highly publicized errors—particularly those that have occurred with children—have highlighted not only the vulnerability of children to the devastating consequences of medication errors, but also the complexity and high risk nature of the medication system that supports pediatric patients. There is a body of evidence that has demonstrated that the rate of error in prescribing medication for hospitalized children is higher than in hospitalized adults.[1,2] Kaushal and colleagues found that the rate of potential adverse drug events in children occurred at a rate three times that in adults.[3] Children's medication doses are typically individualized and based on body weight. Investigators have shown that medication error rates for weight-based dosing are 10.3% versus 5.9% for non-weight based doses.[4]

The emergency department (ED) is a unique clinical care environment. Acuity and volume levels can fluctuate dramatically, patients who present for care are typically unknown to care providers, and variations in patient acuity can result in fragmented care with frequent interruptions and multiple distractions. These factors, combined with the growing prevalence of overcrowding, make the ED a very challenging clinical environment for providers and patients of all ages.[5]

Non-pediatric hospitals will find that a large percentage of their ED patient population is comprised of children, averaging close to 27% nationwide. Even with this significant percentage, many ED staff will attest that they are not comfortable caring for the acutely ill or injured pediatric patient. The root cause for this reduced comfort level (in contrast to adult patient care) can be found in limited training and ongoing experience in caring for acutely/emergently ill children. As an example, nearly 90% of pediatric patient ED visits occur in non-children's hospital settings, with a quarter of those visits occurring in rural hospital EDs that see less than 1,000 children per year.[6] As the vast majority of pediatric patients presenting for care are not severely ill, these factors result in limited ongoing experience in the care of pediatric emergencies for ED staff.

The 2006 Institute of Medicine report, *Emergency Care for Children: Growing Pains,* highlighted many of these concerns, using the word "uneven" to describe the current status of the nation's pediatric emergency care.[7] The report noted that most general hospitals do not require specialized pediatric training for their ED clinical staff. The report also noted that only 6% of U.S. hospitals were equipped with all of the appropriate pediatric resuscitation equipment and medications as recommended in a 2001 policy statement co-authored by the American Academy of Pediatrics and the American College of Emergency Physicians.[8] Similar issues have been raised about ED preparedness for trauma, which is the leading cause of death and disability in children.[9]

Medication systems that support the ED are often different than those that support the inpatient unit. The typical processes that support medication safety for inpatients (unit dose drug distribution systems, pharmacist review of medication orders, pharmacy preparation of complex medication products) are often not part of ED medication systems. Not surprisingly, there is a high rate of medication errors in the ED. It has been reported that there are 100 prescribing errors and 39 administration errors for every 1,000 pediatric patients seen in the ED.[10] One study found that twenty-two percent of acetaminophen orders are written incorrectly for children in this setting.[10] So it seems that there is a "perfect storm" potential when this vulnerable patient that requires complex medication dosing and administration considerations is being treated in an environment that may be sub-optimally equipped to care for children, staffed by providers with limited ongoing experience in caring for critically ill or injured children, and a setting that may have a medication system that does not include some of the safeguards in place for other hospital units.

This chapter identifies key pediatric medication safety concepts, outlines the issues and appropriate methods of medication reconciliation, preparation, and administration, examines the role of both the pharmacist and technology in medication administration, and offers guidelines on the safe sedation practices in pediatric patients.

Medication Reconciliation

As discussed in previous chapters, health care organizations, particularly EDs, must insist on reconciling all medications that children are taking. In bringing focus to the importance of medication reconciliation, the Joint Commission has identified medication reconciliation as one of its National Patient Safety Goals. This goal is described in Sidebar 4-1. In 2009, the Joint Commission announced its intent to review and refine expectations for the medication reconciliation National Patient Safety Goal 8. Until those clarifications are specified by the Joint Commission, surveyors' findings of compliance to NPSG 8 will not contribute to an organization's accreditation score, nor will surveyors' findings generate a Requirement for Improvement (RFI) or appear on the organization's accreditation report. However, surveyors will continue to evaluate compliance with NPSG 8, and organizations are expected to continue to address medication reconciliation across the continuum of care.

Medication reconciliation requires effective communication regarding medication use among numerous people of varying disciplines in multiple locations over time, including the families themselves. One possible workflow consists of the following steps:

- The home medication list is developed.

- The physician reviews this information and makes a decision on each medication.

Sidebar 4-1

2010 National Patient Safety Goal 8*:
Accurately and completely reconcile medications across the continuum of care.

NPSG.08.01.01

A process exists for comparing the patient's current medications with those ordered for the patient while under the care of the hospital.

NPSG.08.02.01

When a patient is referred to or transferred from one hospital to another, the complete and reconciled list of medications is communicated to the next provider of service, and the communication is documented. Alternatively, when a patient leaves the hospital's care to go directly to his or her home, the complete and reconciled list of medications is provided to the patient's known primary care provider, the original referring provider, or a known next provider of service.

Note: When the next provider of service is unknown or when no known formal relationship is planned with a next provider, giving the patient and, as needed, the family, the list of reconciled medications is sufficient.

NPSG.08.03.01

When a patient leaves the hospital's care, a complete and reconciled list of the patient's medications is provided directly to the patient and, as needed, the family, and the list is explained to the patient and/or family.

NPSG.08.04.01

In settings where medications are used minimally or prescribed for a short duration, modified medication reconciliation processes are performed.

Note: This requirement does not apply to hospitals that do not administer medications. It may be important for health care organizations to know which types of medications their patients are taking because these medications could affect the care, treatment, and services provided.

* Based on the 2010 National Patient Safety Goals for Hospitals. For current wording, consult your comprehensive accreditation manual.

Source: The Joint Commission. © 2010.

- The medication orders are written.

- A pharmacist also reviews the home medication list and compares this list with the new medications ordered.

- The pharmacist identifies and resolves any discrepancies between the list and new set of medication orders.

In following an established uniform practice, medication reconciliation is a tool that can help bridge gaps that occur at transitions and transfers of care. Special provisions exist for EDs and other settings where medication use is minimal. These provisions acknowledge that there is often minimal medication use in these settings. Generally new prescriptions are for medications that are used for a short time and do not become part of the patient's chronic regimen. National Patient Safety Goal 08.04.01, as outlined in Sidebar 4-1 above, states that a discharge medication list does not need to be provided if there is no change to home medications following an ED visit. If a short-term medication is prescribed for the patient to take at home, only a list containing that specific medication is required. A comprehensive (or full) discharge home medication list that identifies all medications the patient is to take must be given to the patient if a change is made to chronic

medications (addition of a new chronic medication or change to an existing chronic medication), if the patient requires the additional information because of confusion or some other circumstance that would require providing a complete list to be taken at home, or if the patient is to be admitted. Although the National Patient Safety Goal 8 does not require EDs to communicate changes to the patient's medications to next providers of care, it is important that families be urged to inform their primary or sub-specialty care provider, or another facility involved in the care of the patient, with important details, including changes in medications, that occurred following a visit to the ED. Particularly with pediatric patients, this step is necessary to ensure medications, care, and/or treatment is continued as needed.

Medication Safety in the ED: Addressing the Fundamentals

As discussed in Chapter 3, improving the environment of care in the ED can enhance the safety and quality of care provided to pediatric patients. As a high acuity, rapid-paced unit where quick clinical decisions are essential, ED staff are often in search of ways to improve workflow and increase patient throughput. This continuing quest for efficiency has been made even more urgent with an increasing prevalence of overcrowding. In turn, staff may also be resistant to changes targeted to improve safety that could slow workflow. In ensuring a safe environment of care for pediatric patients it is essential that ED staff operate within a culture that discourages shortcuts that bypass safety nets in efforts to save time. While maintaining their pursuit of more efficient practices, ED staff must adhere to established policies, procedures, and health care standards that emphasize quality and safety as a priority in care delivery.

It is important that staff be aware of the principles and standards that support safe medication use in this hectic environment. Medication storage must be guaranteed to provide security and meet temperature conditions that support product integrity. In the frenzy of the ED environment, automated dispensing machines (ADMs) are widely used as a storage and billing device for medications. They allow for efficient access to medications and tracking of utilization. They have also been proposed to decrease medication errors.[11]

The use of ADMs, however, may lead to shortcuts or workarounds.[11] Most EDs have only one ADM, which is stationary. To save time and steps, ED clinicians may be tempted to use portable carts on which to place patient medications instead of making trips back and forth from the bedside to the ADM. Although this practice does save time, it represents a workaround that bypasses the safety features built into the ADM system. This workaround increases the risk of pulling the wrong medication out of the cart if the patient is receiving look-alike medications, it increases the potential to select one patient's medications for another if more than one patient's medications are placed on the cart and may compromise security of medications as well as optimal storage conditions.[11] EDs should have policies in place to prevent such errors and a culture that prohibits potentially unsafe practices, except for times when this is impractical, such as during resuscitation and other acute patient treatment and stabilization. Safety must always come first, prioritized ahead of convenience or efficiency. Planning for the use of technology that provides ready access to medication, such as ADMs, must also address workflows with that technology that prevent unsafe medication practices.

Allergies: Critical Information

Identifying children's allergies to certain medications is critical to their safety in the ED. According to a recent study, there are significant gaps in the quality and management of information related to medication allergies in the ED setting. Researchers found errors in medication allergy identification introduced at triage that persisted through the care process despite subsequent interactions and data gathering by other ED clinical personnel.[12] Allergies to ingredients that may be found in medications or their packaging, such as eggs or latex, must be captured as part of a thorough allergy history. Many allergies, such as latex, can prove to be fatal. Families should be encouraged to keep records of allergy information for all members of their family. It is also important to determine if the family has been providing the child herbal preparations or other nutraceuticals that could affect the choice or effectiveness of any prescribed medications.

In conducting a patient assessment in the ED, and gaining an accurate medical history, clinicians must identify known allergies in pediatric patients and consider potential, undiagnosed allergies as well. This requires effective communication with the patient, their family, other ED clinicians and other health care providers in the community, including the patient's medical home. The ED should consider and have treatment available for the unanticipated allergic reaction that may manifest itself at any point during the ED visit.

Requirements for Labeling of Medications

Medications need to be properly labeled if they are not given immediately, whether they come from the pharmacy or are prepared in the ED or in another patient care setting. The Joint Commission addresses this issue within the Medication Management standards as well as in Goal 3 of its National Patient Safety Goals, 03.04.01, which requires organizations to label all medications, medication containers (for example, syringes, medicine cups, basins), or other solutions on and off the sterile field in operating rooms or wherever procedures are performed.

Labels should clearly express all pertinent information required for verification of contents by other health care professionals. Auxiliary labels should also be used in situations where they might emphasize an important aspect of the product, such as "For External Use" or "Keep Refrigerated." It is critically important to educate ED staff about the importance of ensuring that medications that are not given immediately are properly labeled with the information required as part of MM.05.01.09 in Sidebar 4-2, page 58. Similarly, syringes and other liquids used in areas where procedures are occurring should be labeled according to the detailed requirements of NPSG 03.04.01, and ED staff should use the information on these labels as part of their performance of the "5 Rights" checking process, which verifies the right patient, right medication, right dose, right route, and right time, prior to administration of the medication.

Safe Medication Prescribing for Children in the ED

Medication prescribing processes are different for children. As medication orders for adult patients are created, the prescriber takes into account typical dosage amounts available for a specific medication and dosing recommendations that are standardized across a variety of adult patient sizes. Pediatric dosing is very different, in that each medication dose and formulations are individualized to the size (and development stage, if applicable) of the child. Prescribers must consider dosing based on milligrams per kilogram of body weight or some variant of this type of equation. Consequently, typical adult dosage formulations for medications will often not accommodate pediatric prescriptions. In a setting that provides care for adults and children, a prescriber will need to employ both dosing techniques. Physicians and other licensed independent practitioners (LIPs) who don't often care for children may not easily remember appropriate pediatric dosing guidelines and may be more prone to make calculation errors. All of these factors can result in prescribing errors for pediatric patients.

Safe prescribing practices in the ED should therefore begin with a policy that requires the measurement and documentation of every pediatric patient's weight in a conspicuous and consistent location in the medical record.[5,13] These measurements should only occur in kilograms. A common and avoidable source of error is the measurement and recording of the child's weight in pounds and ounces, or errors made in converting such measurements to kilograms. Scales that offer measurements in either kilograms or pounds should be replaced by those that offer only results in kilograms. For children who cannot be weighed, EDs should have a readily available tool, such as a length-based dosing guide (e.g., Broselow tape) to assist in the estimation of an accurate weight.

Prescribing practices that support safe medication use are equally if not more important with pediatric medication orders. The use of abbreviations should be avoided, and unacceptable abbreviations identified as part of the Joint Commission's Information Management Standard should be prohibited. As part of this standard, there are requirements for the use of a zero, which is pertinent to pediatric medication orders, as they often require the use of decimal points and zeros. Zeros that trail a decimal point (e.g. 1.0) are dangerous because the decimal point may not be evident and a tenfold dose can be given. In contrast, a preceding zero is absolutely needed before a decimal point (e.g. 0.1) to highlight the presence of the decimal and the fact that the dose is less than a whole integer.

Strategies that support safe medication use in the ED setting must address the risk associated with prescribing for the pediatric patient. Weight-based dosing strategies are typically followed in children under 16 years of age and for those that weigh less than 50 kilograms. When medication doses are derived from a formula that includes a dosing recommendation based on patient body weight, the entire dosing logic should be part of the medication order. As an example, an order for cefazolin would be displayed as follows:

"Cefazolin 50 mg/kg/day x 10 kg = 500 mg/day, divided into 3 doses = 167 mg every 8 hours"

This prescribing practice allows clinicians who have a role in performing a check on the original prescription to see how the dose was created. If the prescriber used the incorrect weight, or made a simple calculation error, this is now identifiable. If the prescriber used a dosing strategy that did not follow recommended dose ranges, it is easily detected when the dosing logic that was used to create the dose is displayed. Certain medications have very broad dosing ranges as defined by multiple clinical indications. This too can be addressed by listing the indicated use for the medication as part of the prescription. Kozer and colleagues found that the use of a formatted medication order sheet, which required the documentation of many of the considerations above, reduced the occurrence of prescribing errors in comparison to a blank order sheet in a pediatric ED.[14]

As hospitals move toward electronic medical records and electronic prescribing, so too do EDs. Hospitals may elect to implement an enterprise-wide EMR system, or an ED-specialty interfaced or stand alone program. Clinical decision support, which provides not only drug-drug interaction, allergy and drug duplication checking, but also upper or lower dosing limits based on weight and age, should be incorporated into any software used to support electronic prescribing of medications. As no single consensus standard for pediatric dosing recommendations yet exists, and as many of the commercial EMR systems will have

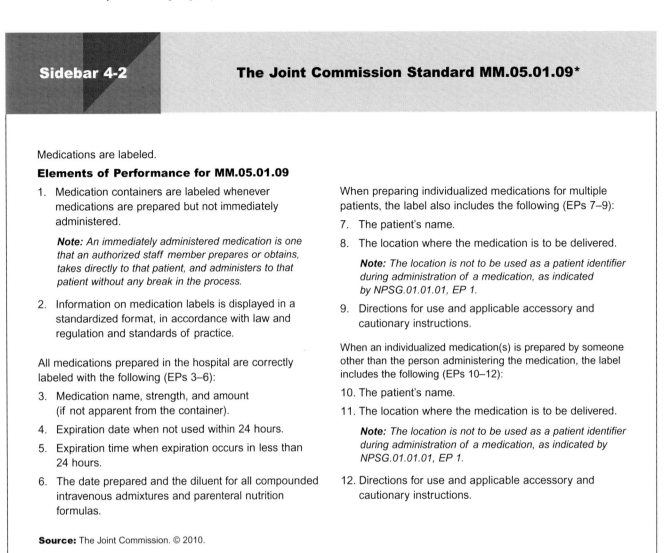

Sidebar 4-2   **The Joint Commission Standard MM.05.01.09***

Medications are labeled.

Elements of Performance for MM.05.01.09

1. Medication containers are labeled whenever medications are prepared but not immediately administered.

    Note: An immediately administered medication is one that an authorized staff member prepares or obtains, takes directly to that patient, and administers to that patient without any break in the process.

2. Information on medication labels is displayed in a standardized format, in accordance with law and regulation and standards of practice.

All medications prepared in the hospital are correctly labeled with the following (EPs 3–6):

3. Medication name, strength, and amount (if not apparent from the container).

4. Expiration date when not used within 24 hours.

5. Expiration time when expiration occurs in less than 24 hours.

6. The date prepared and the diluent for all compounded intravenous admixtures and parenteral nutrition formulas.

When preparing individualized medications for multiple patients, the label also includes the following (EPs 7–9):

7. The patient's name.

8. The location where the medication is to be delivered.

    Note: The location is not to be used as a patient identifier during administration of a medication, as indicated by NPSG.01.01.01, EP 1.

9. Directions for use and applicable accessory and cautionary instructions.

When an individualized medication(s) is prepared by someone other than the person administering the medication, the label includes the following (EPs 10–12):

10. The patient's name.

11. The location where the medication is to be delivered.

    Note: The location is not to be used as a patient identifier during administration of a medication, as indicated by NPSG.01.01.01, EP 1.

12. Directions for use and applicable accessory and cautionary instructions.

Source: The Joint Commission. © 2010.

developed their own provider-support tools, ED and hospital clinical leadership will need to carefully evaluate these tools to assure that they align with local standards for pediatric care.[5] Finally, the presence of pediatric decision support tools does not assure that prescribing clinicians will routinely adopt the guidance offered by these resources. One study evaluating the implementation of computerized order entry found that physicians followed recommendations offered only one-third of the time.[15]

Focusing on Safety in Medication Preparation and Administration

The ED setting is remarkable for having a medication system that often does not have the traditional checks and balances in place that support the medication system in other hospital care units. Due to the acuity and pace of ED patient care and the urgent need for medications, medication preparation often occurs in the ED rather than in the pharmacy. The Joint Commission standards requiring

a pharmacist to review medication orders except for an urgently needed medication or if an LIP is present during administration provides even more relaxed interpretation of these exceptions in this setting.* Hospitals are increasingly recognizing the risk potential of medications prepared in the patient care unit versus the pharmacy and are shifting the system for non-urgent medications to the pharmacy for pharmacist review and preparation. However, in the ED setting, medications are often prepared without pharmacy involvement, which presents a risk for error. The added complexity of preparing pediatric medication doses further increases this risk and particularly in institutions with limited numbers of pediatric visits and the opportunity to practice pediatric medication prescribing, preparation, and administration skills.

---

* Based on The Joint Commission's 2010 *Comprehensive Accreditation Manual for Hospitals*. For current wording, consult your comprehensive accreditation manual.

In the ED, multiple distractions alone can make the preparation and administration of medications a difficult challenge. In one study, nurses were interrupted approximately six times per hour during their shift, and most interruptions occurred while nurses were performing interventions, particularly medication administration.[16] Such interruptions create opportunities for the occurrence of preventable medication errors. Additionally, frequent pages to residents and attending physicians can have a similar effect on the prescribing side. A systematic approach that minimizes distractions in the medication ordering and administration processes should be considered.[17]

Proper medication administration involves a complex set of steps, including precise motor skills, calculation math skills, primary and working memory, attention, focus, and concentration. Studies have determined that medication dosing in children is a particularly high-risk activity, primarily as each dose needs to be tailored to the patient.[18] Medication formulations necessary to achieve these doses are often not commercially available and extemporaneous preparations may need to be created to deliver these doses. This all adds up to a greater level of complexity needed to deliver medications to children.[19]

The act of calculating dosing equations has been identified as a high-error activity, and several factors compound the risk of error when medications are given emergently.[20] All patients should be weighed in kilograms at admission, and their weight should be documented in a consistent location on the patient's chart and on all ED medication orders and home-going prescriptions.

There are limited opportunities for reviews of prescriptions or double-checking, and, in some cases, the inherent stress of managing a life-or-death situation can lead to errors.[5] Tools that help clinicians to quickly assess patients, select appropriate medication doses and sizes of equipment, and monitor patients during resuscitation efforts have the potential to improve patient outcomes. During such critical events, these tools can provide needed information quickly and reduce reliance on memory and error-prone calculations at a time when clinicians are stressed and prone to distractions. Tools such as length-based tapes for pediatric patients can be used to estimate weight and provide precalculated medication doses and can also assist in the selection of appropriate sized equipment. Studies have demonstrated improved accuracy and efficiency for critical decisions in simulated pediatric resuscitations using these tools.[20,21]

Using a Length-Based Tape in Pediatric Treatment

Length-based tapes are used by some ED clinicians to determine the correct dosage of medications and size of key equipment (such as endotracheal tubes, suction catheters) for children. This process can help simplify some of the decision-making in an emergency by eliminating the need to remember the appropriate size tube or medication dose, or the need to accurately estimate a child's weight, which is typically used to calculate the correct dosage for most medications. The ability to recall these facts may be especially challenged during the urgency of resuscitation.

Accurate medication administration to a pediatric patient involves many steps. To provide the proper medication dosage to a child, the practitioner must know the child's weight in kilograms, the milligram dose per kilogram, and the available concentrations of the specific drug. Pediatric resuscitation drugs are not used often enough by most ED clinicians to recall correct medication dosages or concentrations, and valuable time is therefore lost in efforts to search for this information. Complex, time-consuming, and error-prone calculations required may include conversion of weight from pounds to kilograms, or computation of a medication dose volume from the chosen mg/kg dose and concentration of the drug. In using a length-based system tool and/or a pre-calculated dosing resource, the practitioner is able to concentrate on more important cognitive decisions required in emergency care. These tools allow for weight estimation and manual dose calculation to be bypassed, providing pre-calculated doses and pre-determined equipment sizes, and have been shown to reduce deviation from recommended medication dosage ranges.[20] However, problems have also been identified with the use of the length-based tape. When the tape is not used often, it has the potential to be used incorrectly. Patients can be measured incorrectly with the tape (they may be measured from the wrong end of the tape), which may result in an incorrect weight and dose determination.[22] Finally, some versions of these tools may not provide the recommended dose in both weight and volume, necessitating a calculation that could be prone to error.

Relying on Pharmacists in the Medication Use Process

Because of their specialized knowledge of medications and their role in medication preparation, safety, and the drug distribution process, pharmacists are in a unique position to help prevent medication errors and ensure appropriate medication administration. It is preferable that pharmacists working with pediatric patients have specialty training or education in pediatric pharmacology. Pharmacists should play a key role in the ED medication delivery system and interact with other members of the health care team to develop, implement, and, when possible, monitor a therapeutic plan to achieve optimal care for each individual patient, making efforts to detect and resolve drug-related problems before they reach the patient. Organizations should integrate pharmacists into the ED team. Sidebar 4-3 describes the ways in which the pharmacist, as a drug information specialist, can support the medication use process.

Another potential role for the pharmacist in the ED is to support the complex preparation of medications during resuscitation events. This resource may be useful in both low pediatric volume general hospital and high volume children's hospital EDs. "Our pharmacists have proven themselves to be invaluable in this role, and help to free up ED clinical staff for other activities." says Sally Reynolds, M.D., Medical Director, Emergency Department, Children's Memorial Hospital, Chicago, Illinois. "The knowledge and skills brought to resuscitation by our pharmacists has helped to improve our efficiency in the delivery of critical medications and reduces error."

In supporting the ED team, pharmacists should be involved in the development of safe processes and can provide counsel to staff on the use of high-alert medications. High-alert medications are drugs that bear a heightened risk of causing significant patient harm when they are used in error. Although mistakes may or may not be more common with these drugs, the consequences of an error with these medications can result in devastating outcomes to all patients, including children. Table 4-1, page 62, provides a list of high-alert medications.

A second set of eyes to perform an independent double check adds a layer of safety to a high risk medication process. This is a system redundancy that requires a second individual to verify the accuracy of the drug therapy prior to administration. The second individual provides a fresh, unbiased review of the work of the first person. If feasible, ED staff should use the pharmacy to prepare non-urgent doses. If medications must be prepared in the ED, consideration should be given to using an independent double-check process for medications prepared in the ED, or for those medications recognized to pose the highest risk to patients.

Look-Alike, Sound-Alike Medications, and Identification of Risks

With the consistent counsel of the pharmacy department, all ED staff should be aware of drug product names, which are easily confused with other drug names or drug products with look-alike packaging, and their potential to lead to harmful medication errors. Unfortunately, many drug names can look or sound like other drug names. Increasingly, pharmaceutical manufacturers and regulatory authorities are taking measures to determine if there are unacceptable similarities between proposed names and products on the market. Factors such as poor handwriting or poorly communicated verbal prescriptions, however, can exacerbate the problem. In 2001, the Joint Commission published a *Sentinel Event Alert* on look-alike and sound-alike (LASA) drug names. Medications that are packaged in a way that look similar to other marketed products also pose a risk for mix-ups. General strategies EDs can employ to reduce the risk of mix-ups include limiting the number of concentrations of a medication stored in the ED and physically separating two look-alike products (or two concentrations of the same medication). When adult and pediatric strengths of medications must both be kept in the ED, they should especially be labeled to differentiate one from the other. Joint Commission Standard MM.01.02.01, which states "The hospital addresses the safe use of look-alike/sound-alike medications," recognizes that health care organizations and practitioners need to be aware of the role drug names play in medication safety. Included under this standard, EP 1 requires hospitals to develop a list of look-alike/sound-alike medications that it stores, dispenses, or administers. Table 4-2, page 64, provides a list of the most problematic look-alike and sound-alike drug names for the ED setting.

An organization's list of look-alike/sound-alike drugs must contain a minimum of 10 drug combinations, which must be selected from the table posted on the Joint Commission website. Organizations should reassess previous choices in light of new information, including the revised list, and selection of replacement or additional pairs as indicated by the results of that assessment. Internal medication data, formulary decisions, and new products may also be factored into the decision.

Using Technology to Enhance Pediatric Medication Safety

There are numerous technologies available to support staff in today's health care system. As discussed at the outset of this chapter, although there are some time-saving elements associated with new technologies such as automated

| Sidebar 4-3 | **The Role of the Pharmacist in the Medication System** |

- Be available regularly in patient care areas to serve as a source of information to other health care professionals regarding current drug therapies and appropriate use of medications.

- Review the original medication order prior to dispensing the medication, unless emergency circumstances dictate otherwise—screening for prescribing errors, allergies, drug and disease interactions, correct dose, and indication. Dosage calculations should be checked against acceptable dosage ranges. The prescriber of any questionable medication order should be contacted for clarification prior to dispensing the medication. Prior to dispensing, the pharmacist should compare the original order with the label and the product being dispensed. Clinical decision support tools within computerized prescriber order entry systems or pharmacist order entry systems can support appropriate medication dosing decisions.

- Research new or unfamiliar medications, uses, or doses.

- Dispense medications for individual patients in a patient-specific, pre-measured, ready-to-administer form whenever possible. When this is not possible due to medication stability reasons, auxiliary labels should be used to clearly communicate preparation instructions prior to administration. Auxiliary labels should also be used in other situations when they will clearly aid in the prevention of errors.

- Carefully document products used and steps and calculations performed in the preparation or manufacture of a drug product. This is a priority for high alert drugs, those that have the greatest consequences of error. For these medications, it is particularly important that an independent double-check be used for all calculations.

- Carefully document all verbal orders received from prescribers as new orders, renewals, or corrections to a new order. The order should be written down immediately and then read back to the prescriber, confirming that the order was written down correctly.

- Ensure that medications arrive in the patient care area in a timely fashion following the receipt of the order. If medication delivery will be delayed for any reason, such as the need to resolve a problem with the order, the nurse caring for the patient should be notified of the delay and the reason.

- Counsel patients and their caregivers, verifying that they understand the name, purpose, route of administration, dose, dose frequency, potential adverse effects, and how adverse effects might be managed for each medication they are receiving.

Adapted from Levine S.R., Cohen M.R., Blanchard N.R., et al.: Guidelines for preventing medication errors in pediatrics. *J Pediatr Pharmacol Ther* 6: 427–443, 2001.

dispensing machines (ADM), it is important to use them in accordance with established safe practices, with vigilance to workarounds and shortcuts used to circumvent those safe practices. Even when these tools are being used appropriately, it is important to review their use considering the potential for medication errors in the pediatric population, as well as for unanticipated negative impacts on key patient care processes that are unique to the ED.

ADMs are designed to enhance efficiencies within the medication system by providing ready access to medications within a secure cabinet that also provides a means of creating a patient charge when a medication is removed. Acknowledging these enhanced features, implementation of this technology may decrease the use of traditional methods that are employed to enhance safety and may actually increase the number of medication errors.[19] As outlined in Sidebar 4-4, page 69, several issues must be in place before ADMs are used.

Improving Care Through CPOE Systems

Many hospitals and health care systems are developing and/or implementing computerized prescriber order entry (CPOE) systems. CPOE systems can provide a useful platform for integrating evidence-based guidelines into clinicians' workflow by providing "just-in-time" treatment advice or decision support tailored to the needs of the individual patient.[5] Often, different processes for ordering

---

TABLE 4-1

High-Alert Medications

Insulin
Common Risk Factors

- Usually part of floor stock, so product selection and dose are not double checked by pharmacists
- Insulin and heparin vials, kept in close proximity to each other on a nursing unit, leading to mix-ups
- Use of "U" as an abbreviation for "units" in orders (which can be confused with "O," resulting in a tenfold overdose)
- Incorrect rates being programmed into an infusion pump

Suggested Strategies

- Establish an independent double-check process whereby one nurse prepares the dose and another nurse reviews it.
- Do not store insulin and heparin near each other.
- Spell out the word "units" instead of "U."
- Build in an independent double check process for programming of infusion pumps with insulin admixtures.

Narcotics and Opiates
Common Risk Factors

- Parenteral narcotics stored in nursing areas as floor stock, so product selection and dose are not double checked by pharmacists
- Confusion between hydromorphone and morphine
- Patient-controlled analgesia (PCA) and infusion pump programming errors

Suggested Strategies

- Limit the narcotics and opiates available in floor stock.
- Educate staff about hydromorphone and morphine mix-ups.
- Implement protocols for independent double checks with programming of PCA pumps and for preparation of narcotic admixtures as well as infusion pump programming.

Injectable Potassium Chloride or Potassium Phosphate Concentrate
Common Risk Factors

- Storing concentrated potassium chloride/phosphate outside of the pharmacy
- Incorrect preparation of potassium chloride/phosphate admixtures extemporaneously

- Failure to properly dilute potassium chloride/phosphate concentrate prior to administration
- Administration of potassium chloride or potassium phosphate at rates that exceed recommended limits

Suggested Strategies

- Remove concentrated potassium chloride/phosphate from floor stock.
- Use commercially available premixed IV solutions.
- Have pharmacy compound custom preparations including these medications.
- Intravenous Anticoagulants (Heparin)

Common Risk Factors

- Similar labeling and packaging among products
- Multi-dose containers
- Confusion between heparin and insulin due to similar measurement units and proximity

Suggested Strategies

- Standardize concentrations and use premixed solutions.
- Limit the number of available concentrations stored on a patient care unit.
- Use only single-dose containers.
- Separate heparin and insulin and remove heparin from the top of medication carts.
- Double-check infusion pump programming.

Concentrated Sodium Chloride Injections above 0.9 percent
Common Risk Factors

- Storing sodium chloride injections (above 0.9 percent) on nursing units
- Large number of concentrations/formulations available, with potential for mix-up
- No double-check system in place

Suggested Strategies

- Remove concentrated sodium chloride (above 0.9%) from nursing units.
- Preparation of customized admixtures requiring sodium chloride should be performed in the pharmacy.
- Double-check pump rate, drug, concentration, and line attachments.

Source: The Joint Commission.

medications exist in the ED setting compared with those on the inpatient care units. A CPOE system developed to support inpatient care may not be useful in the ED because it may not support ED workflow. Hospitals may need to choose a separate CPOE system for use in the ED setting or may continue to use paper processes to order medications for certain high acuity situations, such as resuscitation. This lack of integration may create opportunities for process failure, which can be addressed through failure mode effects analysis (FMEA) or other proactive risk assessment techniques.

The selection and programming of a computer system should be done with medication error prevention in mind. While CPOE systems appear to reduce medication error rates, it remains unclear as to whether they are consistently effective in reducing adverse events and whether they are associated with improved clinical outcomes. It is important to note, however, that unanticipated problems may result from implementation of a CPOE system, and particularly one that is not customized for children, or for the ED setting. ED clinical managers should consider the unique needs of ED workflow and pediatric patient populations as they evaluate CPOE systems, and in the planning for their implementation, and evaluate the impact of these systems upon ED care delivery, quality, and patient safety.[23] As outlined in Sidebar 4-5, page 70, a variety of functions should be incorporated into the "ideal" computer order entry system.[24]

The use of CPOE and/or approved and preprinted order sets that are based on evidence-based practice should be used to the maximum extent possible to eliminate verbal ordering. Verbal ordering is a potential source for medication error and should be avoided whenever possible. Policies and procedures should be established to require a "read back" technique and should specify circumstances acceptable for verbal orders and personnel permitted to either give or accept this type of order.

Utilizing Smart Pumps and Syringe Pumps in Safe Medication Administration

Another advance in technology that can support ED staff in medication administration are smart pumps. According to the Institute of Medicine Report, *To Err is Human: Building a Safe Health System,* infusion-related errors are associated with the greatest risk of harm, and "smart" (computerized) infusion systems currently are available that alert the user when doses or infusion rates exceed pre-set upper limits.[25]

Smart pumps are designed to promote safe medication administration and prevent errors. These pumps are equipped with features such as a drug library that contains dosing limits and supports accurate dosing (weight based and non-weight based) of medications. The drug library can be customized to match a hospital's particular pharmacy formulary. This feature helps decrease the risk of medication errors when calculating and setting up certain medication infusions.[5] The smart pump is one technological advance that can provide pediatric-specific safeguards if a drug library that includes pediatric-specific dosing limits and pediatric-appropriate standardized concentrations is developed. This technology is available in pumps that are used for adults and pediatric patients.

The syringe pump can deliver very small quantities of medication over a long period. This feature is important to the pediatric population because it easily allows for medication to be delivered in much smaller doses. Additionally, the syringe pump has the capability to deliver precise and regulated infusion rates, which is critical in facilitating more precise therapeutic drug monitoring.[5]

Prescribing Home-Going Medications from the ED

The most frequent source of medication error occurs during the writing of the medication order or prescription. Studies have distinguished the rate of errors in prescriptions within the pediatric ED setting. Upon review of 358 prescriptions provided by ED prescribers to pediatric patients, Taylor et al., noted that 59% contained at least one error.[26] Errors included minor omission of information, incomplete instructions (which was often clarified within the discharge instructions), dose and direction errors, and unclear dispensing quantity. These researchers noted that the rate of error was higher for prescribers who treated both adults and children (such as family practice physicians, emergency medicine physicians, or physicians in training who were completing an internal medicine/pediatrics residency). Rinke and colleagues from Johns Hopkins found that 12.5% of inpatient medication orders for pediatric patients and 4.3% of outpatient prescriptions issued for pediatric patients contained an error.[27] The most common error type was incorrect dose, caused most often by a calculation error and an erroneous weight-based dose target. Their results also showed that those who prescribed less often were more likely to have errors in their prescriptions or inpatient orders. These authors recommended focused education for those who write orders less frequently and generalized interventions focused on techniques to enhance the safety

TABLE 4-2

Look-Alike, Sound-Alike Drug Names

Potential Problematic Drug Names	Brand Name(s) (UPPERCASE) & Generic (lowercase)	Potential Errors and Consequences	Specific Safety Strategies**
1. Concentrated liquid morphine products vs. conventional liquid morphine concentrations	Concentrated: **ROXANOL** morphine oral liquid (conventional concentration)	Concentrated forms of oral morphine solution (20 mg/mL) have often been confused with the conventional concentrations (listed as 10 mg/ 5 mL or 20 mg/5 mL), leading to serious errors. Accidental selection of the wrong concentration, and prescribing/labeling the product by volume, not milligrams, contributes to these errors, some of which have been fatal. For example, "10 mg" has been confused with "10 mL." If concentrated product is used, this represents a 20-fold overdose.	Dispense concentrated oral morphine solutions only when ordered for a specific patient (not as unit stock). Segregate the concentrated solution from the other concentrations wherever it is stored. Purchase and dispense concentrated solutions in dropper bottles (available from at least two manufacturers) to help prevent dose measurement errors and differentiate the concentrated product from the conventional products. Verify that patients and caregivers understand how to measure the proper dose for self-administration at home. For inpatients, dispense concentrated solutions in unit-doses.
2. ephedrine and epinephrine	**ADRENALIN** (epinephrine) ephedrine	The names of these two medications look very similar, and their clinical uses make storage near each other likely, especially in obstetrical areas. Both products are available in similar packaging (1 mL amber ampuls and vials).	See general recommendations below.
3. hydromorphone injection and morphine injection	DILAUDID (hydromorphone) **ASTRAMOPRH, DURAMORPH, INFUMORPH** (morphine)	Some health care providers have mistakenly believed that hydro-morphone is the generic equiva-lent of morphine. However, these products are not interchange-able. Fatal errors have occurred when hydromorphone was con-fused with morphine. Based on equianalgesic dose conversion, this may represent significant overdose, leading to serious ad-verse events. Storage of the two medications in close proximity to one another and in similar con-centrations may contribute to such errors. Confusion has re-sulted in episodes of respiratory arrest due to potency differences between these drugs.	Stock specific strengths for each product that are dissimilar. For example, stock units with hydromorphone 1 mg unit dose cartridges, and morphine in 2 mg unit dose cartridges. Ensure that health care providers are aware that these two products are not interchangeable.

(Continued on next page)

TABLE 4-2

Look-Alike, Sound-Alike Drug Names *(continued)*

Potential Problematic Drug Names	Brand Name(s) (UPPERCASE) & Generic (lowercase)	Potential Errors and Consequences	Specific Safety Strategies**
4. *hydroxyzine and hydralazine*	**VISTARIL, ATARAX** (hydroxyzine)	Because the first four letters of their names are identical, they are frequently stored next to one another on pharmacy shelves and automated dispensing cabinets and listed adjacently on computer screens. Their similar dosage strengths (10, 25, 50 and 100 mg) and tablet dosage forms also contribute to confusion. Confusion between the antihistamine (hydroxyzine) and the antihypertensive agent (hydralazine) could lead to serious adverse drug events.	Change appearance of look-alike product names on computer screens, pharmacy and nursing unit shelf labels and bins (including automated dispensing cabinets), pharmacy product labels, and medication administration records. Differentiate drug names by using boldface, color, and/or "tall man" letters, to help emphasize the letter characters in each name that are unique to that name (e.g., hydrOXYzine, hydrALAzine). Choose generic manufacturers whose products exhibit clear labeling with "tall man" characters.
5. Insulin products Humalog and Humulin Novolog and Novolin Humulin and Novolin Humalog and Novolog Novolin 70/30 and Novolog Mix 70/30	**HUMULIN** (human insulin products) **HUMALOG** (insulin lispro) **NOVOLIN** (human insulin products) **NOVOLOG** (human insulin aspart) **NOVOLIN** 70/30 (70% isophane insulin [NPH] and 30% insulin injection [regular]) **NOVOLOG MIX** 70/30 (70% insulin aspart protamine suspension and 30% insulin aspart)	Similar names, strengths and concentration ratios of some products (e.g. 70/30) have contributed to medication errors. Mix-ups have also occurred between the 100 unit/mL and 500 units/mL insulin concentrations.	Limit the use of insulin analog 70/30 mixtures to just a single product. Limit the variety of insulin products stored in patient care units, and remove patient-specific insulin vials from stock upon discharge. For drug selection screens, emphasize the word "mixture" or "mix" along with the name of the insulin product mixtures. Consider auxiliary labels for newer products to differentiate them from the established products. Also apply bold labels on atypical insulin concentrations.

(Continued on next page)

TABLE 4-2

Look-Alike, Sound-Alike Drug Names *(continued)*

Potential Problematic Drug Names	Brand Name(s) (UPPERCASE) & Generic (lowercase)	Potential Errors and Consequences	Specific Safety Strategies**
6. Lipid-based daunorubicin and doxorubicin products vs. conventional forms of daunorubicin and doxorubicin	**Lipid-based:** **DOXIL** (doxorubicin liposomal) **DAUNOXOME** (daunorubicin citrate liposomal) **Conventional:** **CERUBIDINE** (daunorubicin, conventional) **ADRIAMYCIN, RUBEX** (doxorubicin, conventional)	Many drugs now come in liposomal formulations indicated for special patient populations. Confusion may occur between the liposomal and the conventional formulation because of name similarity. The products are not interchangeable. Lipid-based formulation dosing guidelines differ significantly from conventional dosing. For example, a standard dose of doxorubicin liposomal is 20 mg/m2 given at 21-day intervals, compared to doses of 50 to 75 mg/m2 every 21 days for conventional drug. Doses of liposomal daunorubicin are typically 40 mg/m2 repeated every two (2) weeks, while doses of conventional daunorubicin vary greatly and may be administered more frequently. Accidental administration of the liposomal form instead of the conventional form has resulted in severe side effects and death.	Staff involved in handling these products should be aware of the differences between conventional and lipid-based formulations of these drugs. Encourage staff to refer to the lipid-based products by their brand names and not just their generic names. Stop and verify that the correct drug is being used if staff, patients, or family members notice a change in the solution's appearance from previous infusions. Lipid-based products may be seen as cloudy rather than a clear solution. Storage of lipid-based products in patient care areas and automated dispensing cabinets is highly discouraged. Include specific method of administration for these products.

(Continued on next page)

TABLE 4-2

Look-Alike, Sound-Alike Drug Names *(continued)*

Potential Problematic Drug Names	Brand Name(s) (UPPERCASE) & Generic (lowercase)	Potential Errors and Consequences	Specific Safety Strategies**
7. Lipid-based amphotericin products vs. conventional forms of amphotericin	**Lipid-based:** **AMBISOME** (amphotericin B liposomal) **ABELCET** (amphotericin B lipid complex) **Conventional:** **AMPHOCIN, FUNGIZONE INTRAVENOUS** (amphotericin B desoxycholate)	Many drugs now come in liposomal formulation indicated for special patient populations. Confusion may occur between the liposomal and the conventional formulations because of name similarity. The products are not interchangeable. Lipid-based formulation dosing guidelines differ significantly from conventional dosing. Conventional amphotercin B desoxycholate doses should not exceed 1.5 mg/kg/day. Doses of the lipid-based products are higher, but vary from product to product. If conventional amphotericin B is given at a dose appropriate for a lipid-based product, a severe adverse event is likely. Confusion between these products has resulted in episodes of respiratory arrest and other dangerous, sometimes fatal outcomes due to potency differences between these drugs.	Staff involved in handling these products should be aware of the differences between conventional and lipid-based formulations of these drugs. Encourage staff to refer to the lipid-based products by their brand names and not just their generic names. Stop and verify that the correct drug is being used if staff, patients or family members notice a change in the solution's appearance from previous infusions. Lipid-based products may be seen as cloudy rather than a clear solution. Storage of lipid-based products in patient care areas and automated dispensing cabinets is highly discouraged. To reduce potential for confusion, consider limiting lipid-based amphotericin B products to one specific brand.
8. *metformin and metronidazole*	**FLAGYL** (metronidazole) **GLUCOPHAGE** (metformin)	Potentially serious mix-ups between metronidazole and metformin have been linked to look-alike packaging (both bulk bottles and unit-dose packages) and selection of the wrong product after entering MET as a mnemonic. Metformin is contraindicated in certain clinical situations where use might contribute to lactic acidosis. Administration of intravenous iodinated contrast media during radiologic procedures has been associated with acute renal dysfunction.	To avoid order entry errors, program computer order entry software to display entire names of associated products whenever the MET stem is used as a mnemonic. Use tall man letters for unique letter characters in names. Pharmacy should consider stocking metronidazole in only 250 mg tablets (metformin tablets are not available as 250 mg tablets.) See also the general recommendations below.

(Continued on next page)

TABLE 4-2

Look-Alike, Sound-Alike Drug Names *(continued)*

Potential Problematic Drug Names	Brand Name(s) (UPPERCASE) & Generic (lowercase)	Potential Errors and Consequences	Specific Safety Strategies**
9. *OxyContin and oxycodone*	**OXYCONTIN** (oxycodone controlled-release) oxycodone (immediate release)	Mix-ups occur when staff confuse brand name, OxyContin, with oxycodone, or the prescriber uses the generic name to order the controlled release formulation without specifying "controlled release." Patient may receive immediate release product in dose appropriate for controlled release. Significant overdose may occur.	Do not store immediate release and controlled release products together. If possible, have the pharmacy dispense oral oxycodone products for individual patients. Always specify dosage form. Use available brand name when prescribing. Educate staff about the potential for confusion. See general recommendations below.
10. vinblastine and vincristine	**VELBAN** (vinblastine) **ONCOVIN** (vincristine)	Fatal errors have occurred, often due to name similarity, when patients were erroneously given vincristine intravenously, but at the higher vinblastine dose. A typical vincristine dose is usually capped at around 1.4 mg/m^2 weekly. The vinblastine dose is variable but, for most adults, the weekly dosage range is 5.5 to 7.4 mg/m^2.	Install maximum dose warnings in computer systems to alert staff to name mix-ups during order entry. Do not store these agents near one another. Staff involved in handling these products should be aware of the differences. Use brand names or brand and generic names when prescribing and do not use abbreviations for these drug names.

* Note: The name pairs listed were selected after a review of error report descriptions received by the Institute for Safe Medication Practices, the United States Pharmacopeia, the U.S. Food and Drug Administration, and the Pennsylvania Patient Safety Reporting System (Pa-PSRS). Ratings based on judgments of severity and likelihood of confusion in the clinical setting were provided by outside experts using a modified Delphi process. The list was updated in August 2006, with deletions or additions recommended by medication safety staff at ISMP, USP, and FDA and also based upon frequency of reports and potential outcome severity. Appreciation is expressed to Medco Health Solutions for their input to the ambulatory drug portion of these listings. The assistance of ISMP in providing potential error consequences and safety strategies for this project is also appreciated.

** These safety strategies are not inclusive of all possible strategies to reduce name-related errors. Also see General Recommendation for Preventing Drug Name Mix-ups available at www.jointcommission.org.

Source: The Joint Commission.

Sidebar 4-4	**Issues to Consider Before ADMs Are Used**

- Although it does not always happen in the ED, consideration should be given to having the ADM interface with the pharmacy computer system and having the pharmacist review the new order prior to allowing access to the drug within the ADM. Although some ADMs send information to the pharmacy system, they do not alert the pharmacy that a medication has been released for administration to a patient.

- For ADMs that are profiled, an override process is often put in place to allow access to a defined list of medications for emergency situations where timely review of the order by the pharmacist may not be possible. The override function must be addressed at the time of implementation and should be restricted to true "emergencies." If a liberal approach is used and the function becomes one of convenience and not one of true urgency, many errors may be allowed to occur prior to pharmacist review. Even during emergencies the pharmacist should be alerted to the incident. As stated above, some systems will send information to the pharmacy system; however, they do not alert the pharmacy that a medication has been released for administration to a patient. Alternatively, during emergencies a second nurse could verify the order before administration to a patient. All overridden reports should be routinely checked for patterns.

- The use of ADMs in the pediatric setting may also decrease the use of patient-specific unit doses. Although these machines may contain commercial unit dose containers, they are not specific to that patient and act as bulk containers. Nurses are required to calculate doses and draw up medications, and another practitioner should verify the dose before administration.

- Medication inventory in each ADM can be tailored to specific patient care units to assure that medications unfamiliar to a practitioner cannot be removed in error. Careful drug selection based on the needs of the patient care unit, patient age, diagnosis, and staff expertise should be used to tailor each ADM.

- Systems that use matrix drawers, which provide access to multiple medications when the drawer is opened, increase the risk of selecting the wrong medication or provide an opportunity for a medication to inadvertently fall into the wrong container. This may be addressed by the use of an ADM with specific cells for each drug that limit selection to only that drug.

- Processes that limit restocking errors in ADMs through the use of double-checks or bar code technology should be employed.

- With the growing utilization of ADMs there are now an increasing number of locations where medications can be stored. Multiple locations may increase the number of missing or non-stocked medications. Missing medications can result in delays for patients and may result in multiple doses being administered.

- Some additional safety recommendations include: (1) minimize variety; (2) stock unit dose drugs in the smallest dose/container size available; (3) supply only a single concentration of a medication; and (4) medication returns should be made to the pharmacy and not to the ADM, unless there is a specific return bin within the ADM dedicated to returned drugs.

Adapted from Pape T.: Workaround error. Agency for Healthcare Research and Quality (AHRQ) Home Page, February 2006, www.ahrq.gov.

Levine S.R., Cohen M.R., Blanchard N.R., et al.: Guidelines for preventing medication errors in pediatrics. *J Pediatr Pharmacol Ther* 6:427–443, 2001.

of prescribing for the pediatric patient.[27] It is important to appreciate the prevalence of errors that occur when prescribing and the importance of using techniques such as showing dosing logic to increase the likelihood of errors being detected by the individual who will perform the next check.

A recognized source of medication errors for all consumers is improper use of medications in the home setting. Although this is a significant public health issue for all members of the public, the very nature of the added complexity of providing medication doses to children increases the risk of error. Simon and Weinkle demonstrated, through the use of mock situations where caregivers were asked to determine and measure the correct dose of acetaminophen for their child, that only 30% of caregivers were able to demonstrate both accurately measured and the correct dose of medication.[28] Frush and colleagues were able to show a higher deviation

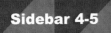

Sidebar 4-5

Functions Important to the "Ideal" Computer Order Entry System

- Prescriber order entry with verification by pharmacist

- Computer-generated medication administration records from a common database shared with the pharmacy and the prescriber

- For each patient, readily accessible lists of current medications are available to caregivers

- Multi-directional interface between the pharmacy and other institutional systems (e.g., laboratory, admission and discharge, clinical records)

- Access to historical patient data (i.e., archived information)

- Ability to calculate and verify appropriate height–weight range and dosage for patient

- Access to vital patient and drug information directly from order entry, medication profile, and medication administration screens

- Ability of system to use patient and drug information as well as software to provide clinical decision support during order entry to reduce potential for adverse drug events (e.g., drug interactions, contraindications, excessive or inadequate doses, allergies). This should be part of a comprehensive decision support program. These programs would include checking for laboratory results and advising the prescriber of the need for dosing modifications for specified medications. Automatic checking should also include medication allergies, drug–drug interactions, drug–nutrient interactions, drug duplication, therapeutic duplication, contraindicated medications, weight-based dosage checking.

- Provide a forced function by limiting the route and frequency by which a drug is ordered

- Require entry of allergy information and patient's weight in kilograms before accepting order

Adapted from: Pape T.: Workaround error. *Agency for Healthcare Research and Quality (AHRQ)* Home Page, February 2006, http://www.webmm.ahrq.gov/case.aspx?caseID=118 (accessed Feb. 16, 2009).

Levine S.R., Cohen M.R., Blanchard N.R., et al.: Guidelines for preventing medication errors in pediatrics. *J Pediatr Pharmacol Ther* 6:427–443, 2001.

from the correct dose calculation and dose measurement in a control group of caregivers versus a group of caregivers who were provided with a color coded method for determining and measuring the correct dose correctly.[29]

Why is there a tendency for error in the provision of medication to pediatric patients? This relates to the issue of health literacy, or the limited capacity of patients and families to follow instructions on prescription bottles, perform calculations, and provide general care for themselves. The challenges of understanding information vital to care for themselves or loved ones are not just pertinent to illiterate consumers. A recent Joint Commission white paper addressed the health literacy problem. Among Americans, literacy is at a basic level for 29% and below basic for 14%. The ability of Americans to use numbers is even lower, with 33% at a basic level and 22% below basic skills. Forty-four percent of Americans are intermediate prose-literate, which means that they can read moderately dense information and break it down to simple conclusions. However, medication instructions, consent forms, and insurance forms can be extremely complex. Health literacy is not just the ability to understand words and numbers: there are social, cultural, and economic components that need to be factored in.

Those who provide health care need to improve their ability to make the patient or caregiver understand, or this communication gap may adversely affect the patients' health outcome. Health care practitioners must become more adept at creating patient's understanding.[30] To help patients and caregivers better understand dosing techniques, pictograms should be considered as a viable teaching tool. Using pictograms to illustrate correct dosing techniques during medication counseling for caregivers of children has shown to increase medication regimen adherence and reduce medication errors.[31] Another important intervention when providing instructions to caregivers is to confirm that the caregiver can demonstrate how to measure the correct dose. Health care providers should ask the caregiver to demonstrate how to measure the dose and to confirm that the correct amount has been drawn up. Consideration should also be given to providing an accurate measure for the dose (household teaspoons are not standardized in size and will often provide inaccurate measures of dosage quantities) in the form of an oral syringe.

Monitoring and Managing Pediatric Sedation and Analgesia

The state-of-the-art practice of pediatric emergency care mandates effective management for pain and anxiety.

Children may require the administration of sedation/analgesia to support the success of necessary diagnostic or therapeutic interventions. The safe sedation of children for procedures requires a systematic approach that also includes the following[32]:

- No administration of sedating medication without the safety net of qualified medical supervision.

- Careful pre-sedation evaluation for underlying medical or surgical conditions that would place the child at increased risk from sedating medications.

- A focused airway examination for anatomic abnormalities that might increase the potential for airway obstruction.

- Appropriate fasting for elective procedures and a balance between depth of sedation and risk for those who are unable to fast because of the urgent nature of the procedure.

- A clear understanding of the pharmacokinetic and pharmacodynamic effects of the medications used for sedation and analgesia, as well as an appreciation for drug interactions.

- Appropriate training and skills in airway management to allow rescue of the patient.

- Presence of age- and size-appropriate equipment for airway management and venous access.

- Availability of appropriate resuscitation medications and reversal agents.

- Sufficient numbers of qualified staff to perform the procedure and monitor the patient. This requires the presence of one staff member whose sole responsibility is to monitor the patient.

- Appropriate physiologic monitoring during and after the procedure until the patient has achieved recovery.

- A properly equipped and staffed recovery area; recovery to presedation level of consciousness before discharge from medical supervision; and appropriate discharge protocols and instructions.

- Delivery of sedation by a provider who is properly credentialed by the organization to do so.

Sedation in children is often administered to mitigate behavior to allow the safe completion of a procedure. A child's ability to control his or her own behavior to cooperate for a procedure depends both on his or her chronologic and developmental age. Another key factor is whether sufficient analgesia has been achieved for painful conditions or invasive procedures. Younger children and those with developmental delay may require deeper levels of sedation to gain control of their behavior. Therefore, the need for deep sedation should be anticipated. Children in this age group are particularly vulnerable to the sedating medication's effects on respiratory drive, patency of the airway, and protective reflexes. Because children can vary in their responses to a specific dose of a specific sedative, practitioners will need the skills to provide airway and ventilation support and cardiovascular management that would be anticipated for the higher level of sedation that was intended.[33] For older children, and more cooperative younger children, other modalities such as parental presence, hypnosis, distraction, topical local anesthetics, and guided imagery, may reduce the need or the depth for pharmacologic sedation.[34]

The American Academy of Pediatrics has issued guidelines for the monitoring and management of pediatric patients during and after sedation. Sidebar 4-6, page 72, contains an excerpt of these guidelines, which includes documentation requirements.

Pain Management

In addition to consideration of sedation needs, management of pain that may result from disease, a diagnostic procedure or a therapeutic procedure must be ensured. Historically, an understanding of the pain management needs of the pediatric patient have not kept pace with the needs of their adult counterparts. Inadequate sedation and pain control have long-standing implications for the pediatric patient, resulting in altered responses to painful experiences well into the future.[35]

Pain should be assessed at the point of triage and then reassessed as indicated throughout the course of care. Assessment is the first step in the adequate management of pain. A self-reporting scale for level of pain can be used for children as young as three years of age. Training in the use of these tools, and tools to assess the presence of distress in infants and developmentally impaired children, should be provided for ED staff. Pain management practices should also embrace family-centered care. Family members can be instrumental in assisting staff in the assessment of pain in children. Pain treatment protocols should be developed that provide both pharmacologic and non-pharmacologic options and recommended doses for established pain medications.[35] Accurate assessment of pain and timely and effective interventions are vital components of high-quality pediatric care and an important driver of patient and family satisfaction.

Sidebar 4-6	Monitoring and Managing Pediatric Patients During and After Sedation: General Guidelines	

The goals of sedation and analgesia in a pediatric patient for diagnostic and therapeutic procedures are to:

(1) guard the patient's safety and welfare;

(2) minimize physical discomfort and pain;

(3) control anxiety, minimize psychological trauma, and maximize the potential for amnesia;

(4) control behavior and/or movement to allow the optimal outcome and safe completion of the procedure; and

(5) return the patient to a state in which safe discharge from medical supervision, as determined by recognized criteria, is possible. Recommended discharge criteria are listed in Table 1.

Table 1: Recommended Discharge Criteria Following Sedation

1. Cardiovascular function and airway patency are satisfactory and stable.

2. The patient is easily arousable, and protective reflexes are intact.

3. The state of hydration is adequate.

4. The patient can talk (if age and patient appropriate).

5. The patient can sit up unaided (if age and patient appropriate).

6. For a very young, medically complex, or severely developmentally delayed child incapable of the usually expected responses, the pre-sedation level of responsiveness or a level as close as possible to the baseline level for that child should be achieved.

Candidates: Patients who are in American Society of Anesthesiologists (ASA) classes I and II, as described in Table 2, are frequently considered appropriate candidates for minimal, moderate, or deep sedation in the ED setting. Children in ASA classes III and IV, children with special health care needs, and those with anatomic airway abnormalities (e.g., extreme tonsillar hypertrophy or macroglossia, Pierre-Robin syndrome) present issues that require additional and individual consideration, particularly for moderate and deep sedation. ED practitioners are encouraged to consult with appropriate pediatric subspecialists and/or an anesthesiologist for patients with an increased risk of experiencing adverse sedation events because of their underlying medical/surgical conditions.

Table 2: ASA Physical Status Classification

Class I	A normally healthy patient
Class II	A patient with mild systemic disease (e.g., controlled reactive airway disease)
Class III	A patient with severe systemic disease (e.g., a child who is actively wheezing)
Class IV	A patient with severe systemic disease that is a constant threat to life (e.g., a child with status asthmaticus)
Class V	A moribund patient who is not expected to survive without the operation (e.g., a patient with cardiomyopathy requiring ongoing medication therapy)

Responsible Person: The pediatric patient should be accompanied to and from the treatment facility by a parent, legal guardian, or other responsible person. It is preferable to have two or more adults accompany children who are still in car safety seats if transportation to and from a treatment facility is provided by one of the adults.

Facilities: The practitioner who uses sedation must have immediately available facilities, personnel, and equipment to manage emergency and rescue situations. The most common serious complications of sedation involve compromise of the airway or depressed respirations resulting in airway obstruction, hypoventilation, hypoxemia, and apnea. Another common complication of sedation is vomiting. Practitioners should be prepared for this during the procedure and while the patient is recovering. As sedated patients can have an altered gag response, this can be hazardous. Vomiting is also a common post-sedation event reported by families.

Hypotension and cardiopulmonary arrest may occur, usually from inadequate recognition and treatment of respiratory compromise. Other rare complications may include seizures and allergic reactions. Facilities that provide pediatric sedation should monitor for, and be prepared to treat, such complications.

Back-up Emergency Services: A protocol for access to back-up emergency services should be clearly identified with an outline of the procedures necessary for immediate use. For non-hospital facilities, a protocol for ready access to ambulance services and immediate activation of the EMS system for life-threatening complications must be established and maintained. It should be understood that the availability of EMS services does not replace the practitioner's responsibility to provide initial rescue in managing life-threatening complications.

(Continued on next page)

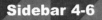

Sidebar 4-6

Monitoring and Managing Pediatric Patients During and After Sedation: General Guidelines
(continued)

On-Site Monitoring and Rescue Equipment:
An emergency cart or kit must be immediately accessible. This cart or kit must contain equipment to provide the necessary age- and size-appropriate drugs and equipment to resuscitate a non-breathing and unconscious child. The contents of the kit must allow for the provision of continuous life support while the patient is being transported to a medical facility or to another area within a medical facility. All equipment and drugs must be checked and maintained on a scheduled basis. Monitoring devices, such as electrocardiography (ECG) machines, pulse oximeters (with size-appropriate oximeter probes), end-tidal carbon dioxide monitors, and defibrillators (with size-appropriate defibrillator paddles), must have a safety and function check on a regular basis as required by local or state regulation.

Documentation: Documentation before sedation shall include, but not be limited to, the guidelines that follow.

- Informed consent: the patient record shall document that appropriate informed consent was obtained according to local, state, and institutional requirements.

- Instructions and information provided to the responsible person: the practitioner shall provide verbal and/or written instructions to the responsible person. Information shall include objectives of the sedation and anticipated changes in behavior during and after sedation.

  - Special instructions shall be given to the responsible adult for infants and toddlers who will be transported home in a car safety seat regarding the need to carefully observe the child's head position to avoid airway obstruction. Transportation in a car safety seat poses a particular risk for infants who have received medications known to have a long half-life, such as chloral hydrate, intramuscular pentobarbital, or a phenothiazine. Consideration for a longer period of observation shall be given if the responsible person's ability to observe the child is limited (only one adult who also has to drive).

  - Another indication for prolonged observation would be a child with an anatomic airway problem or a

severe underlying medical condition. A 24-hour telephone number for the practitioner or his or her associates shall be provided to all patients and their families. Instructions shall include limitations of activities and appropriate dietary precautions.

Dietary Precautions: As mentioned earlier, agents used for sedation have the potential to impair protective airway reflexes, particularly during deep sedation. Although a rare occurrence, pulmonary aspiration may occur if the child regurgitates and cannot protect his or her airway. Therefore, it is prudent that before sedation, the practitioner evaluate preceding food and fluid intake. It is likely that the risk of aspiration during procedural sedation differs from that during general anesthesia involving tracheal intubation or other airway manipulation. However, because the absolute risk of aspiration during procedural sedation is not yet known, guidelines for fasting periods before elective sedation should generally follow those used for elective general anesthesia. For emergency procedures in children who have not fasted, the risks of sedation and the possibility of aspiration must be balanced against the benefits of performing the procedure promptly. Additional research is needed to better elucidate the relationships between various fasting intervals and sedation complications.

Competency: Anyone providing elective or emergent sedation and analgesia for children or performing an invasive procedure, for which the sedation/analgesia is intended to support, should be competent to do so. ED clinical managers, in concert with the hospital medical staff leadership, should define these competencies and their related expectations.

Although not specifically required by the Joint Commission, considering the potential risks associated with sedation of pediatric patients, particularly in EDs with low pediatric patient volumes and limited opportunities to provide this service, the addition of a time-out exercise prior to the initiation of sedation may serve to further enhance patient safety, for both sedation and the procedure it supports.

Adapted from American Academy of Pediatrics, American Academy of Pediatric Dentistry: Cote C.J., Wilson S., Work Group on Sedation. Guidelines for monitoring and management of pediatric patients during and after sedation for diagnostic and therapeutic procedures: an update. *Pediatrics* 118(6):2587–2602, 2006. Printed with permission.

ASA Physical Status Classification System. http://www.asahq.org/clinical/physicalstatus.htm (accessed Jul. 17, 2009).

References

1. Bates D.W., Boyle D.L., Vander Vliet M.B., et al.: *J Gen Intern Med* 10:199–205, 1995.
2. Marino B.L., Reinhardt K., Eichelberger W.J., et al.: Outcomes Manag Nurs Pract 4:129–135, 2000.
3. Khaushal R., Bates D.W., Landrigan C., et al.: Medication errors and adverse drug events in pediatric inpatients. *JAMA* 285:2114–20, 2001.
4. Herout P.M., Erstad B.L.: Impact of computerized physician order entry in the ICU. *Crit Care Med* 32(2):428–32, 2004.
5. Frush K., Krug S., and the American Academy of Pediatrics Committee on Pediatric Emergency Medicine: Patient safety in the pediatric emergency care setting. *Pediatrics* 120:1367–1375, Dec. 2007 (doi:10.1542/peds.2007–2902).
6. Gausche-Hill M., Schmitz C., Lewis R.J.: Pediatric preparedness of United States emergency departments: a 2003 survey. *Pediatrics* 120:1229–1237, 2007.
7. Institute of Medicine, Committee on the Future of Emergency Care in the United States Health System: *Emergency care for children: growing pains.* Washington, D.C.: National Academies Press, 2006.
8. American Academy of Pediatrics, Committee on Pediatric Emergency Medicine and American College of Emergency Physicians, Pediatric Committee: Care of children in the emergency department: guidelines for preparedness. *Pediatrics* 107(4):777–781, 2001.
9. Tuggle D., Krug S., American Academy of Pediatrics Section on Orthopaedics, Committee on Pediatric Emergency Medicine, Section on Critical Care, Section on Surgery, Section on Transport Medicine, Pediatric Orthopaedic Society Of North America: Management of pediatric trauma. *Pediatrics* 121(4):849–854, 2008.
10. Aspden P., Wolcott J., Bootman J.L., et al.: Preventing Medication Errors: *Quality Chasm Series.* Washington, D.C.: National Academy Press, 2007.
11. Pape T.: *Workaround Error.* Agency for Healthcare Research and Quality (AHRQ) Home Page, February 2006, http://www.webmm.ahrq.gov/case.aspx?caseID=118 (accessed Nov. 29, 2007).
12. Porter S.C., Manzi S.F., Volpe D., Stack A.M.: Getting the data right: information accuracy in pediatric emergency medicine. *Quality Safety Healthcare* 15:296–301, 2006.
13. Gausche-Hill M., Krug S.E., and the American Academy of Pediatrics Committee on Pediatric Emergency Medicine, American College of Emergency Physicians Pediatric Committee, Emergency Nurses Association Pediatric Committee: Guidelines for care of children in the emergency department. *Pediatrics* 124:1233–1243, Oct. 2009.
14. Kozer E., Scolnick D., MacPherson A., et al.: Using a preprinted order sheet to reduce prescription errors in a pediatric emergency department: a randomized, controlled trial. *Pediatrics* 116:1299–1302, 2005.
15. Killea B.K., Kaushal R., Cooper M., Kuperman G.J.: To what extent do pediatricians accept computer-based dosing suggestions? *Pediatrics* 119:e69–e75, 2007.
16. Potter P., Wolf L., Boxerman S., et al.: Understanding the cognitive work of nursing in the acute care environment. *J Nurs Admin* 35:327–335, 2005.
17. Fox G.N.: Minimizing prescribing errors in infants and children. Am Fam Phys; Mar 53(4):1319–1325, 1996.
18. Fortescue E.B., Kaushal R., Landrigan C.P., et al.: Prioritizing strategies for preventing medication errors and adverse drug events in pediatric inpatients. *Pediatrics* 111(4 Pt. 1):722–729, 2003.
19. Levine S.R., Cohen M.R., Blanchard N.R., et al.: Guidelines for preventing medication errors in pediatrics. *J Pediatr Pharmacol Ther* 6:427–443, 2001.
20. Shah A.N., Frush K., Luo X., et al.: Effect of an intervention standardized system on pediatric dosing and equipment size determination: a crossover trial involving simulated resuscitation events. *Arch Pediatr Adolesc Med* 157(3):220–236, 2003.
21. Frush K., Hohenhaus S., Luo X., et al.: Evaluation of a web-based education program on reducing medication dosing error. *Pediatr Emerg Care* 22:62–70, 2006.
22. Hohenhaus S.M., Frush K.S.: Pediatric patient safety: common problems in the use of resuscitative aids for simplifying pediatric emergency care. *J Emerg Nurs* 30(1):49–51, 2004.
23. Handler J.A., Feied C.F., Coonan K., et al.: Computerized physician order entry and online decision support. *Acad Emerg Med* 11:1135–1141, 2004.
24. Morgan N., Luo X., Fortner C., et al.: Opportunities for performance improvement in relation to medication administration during pediatric stabilization. *Quality Safety Health Care* 15:179–183, Jun. 2006.
25. Institute of Medicine: *To err is human: building a safer health system.* Washington, D.C.: National Academy Press, 1999.
26. Taylor B.L., Selbst S.M., Shah A.E.: Prescription writing errors in the pediatric emergency department. *Pediatr Emerg Care* 21(12):822–827, 2005.
27. Rinke M.L., Moon M., Clark J.S., et al.: Prescribing errors in a pediatric emergency department. *Pediatric Emergency Care* 24(1):1–8, 2008.
28. Simon H.K., Weinkle D.A.: Over-the-counter medications. *Arch Pediatr Adolesc Med* 151:634–636, 1997.
29. Frush K.S., Luo X., Hutchinson P., et al.: Evaluation of a method to reduce over-the-counter medication dosing error. *Arch Pediatr Adolesc Med* 158:620–624, 2004.
30. "What did the doctor say?" *Improving Health Literacy to Protect Patient Safety.* The Joint Commission, 2007.
31. Yin H.S., Dreyer B.P., van Schaick L., et al.: Randomized controlled trial of a pictogram-based intervention to reduce liquid medication dosing errors and improve adherence among caregivers of young children. *Arch Pediatr Adolesc Med* 162:814–822, Sep. 2008.
32. Committee on Drugs, American Academy of Pediatrics. Guidelines for monitoring and management of pediatric patients during and after sedation for diagnostic and therapeutic procedures: addendum. *Pediatrics* 110(4):836–838, 2002.
33. Mace S.E., Brown L.A., Francis L., et al.: Clinical policy: critical issues in the sedation of pediatric patients in the emergency department. *Ann Emerg Med*; 51(4):378–399, 2008.
34. Cote C.J., Wilson S., Work Group on Sedation, American Academy of Pediatrics, American Academy of Pediatric Dentistry: Guidelines for monitoring and management of pediatric patients during and after sedation for diagnostic and therapeutic procedures: an update. *Pediatrics* 118(6):2587–2602, 2006 PMID: 17142550.
35. Zempsky W.T., Cravero J.P., Committee on Pediatric Emergency Medicine and Section on Anesthesiology and Pain Medicine, American Academy of Pediatrics: Clinical report: relief of pain and anxiety in pediatric patients in emergency medical systems. *Pediatrics* 114(5):1348–1356, 2004.

CHAPTER 5

Infection Prevention and Control Issues Unique to Pediatric Patients in the ED

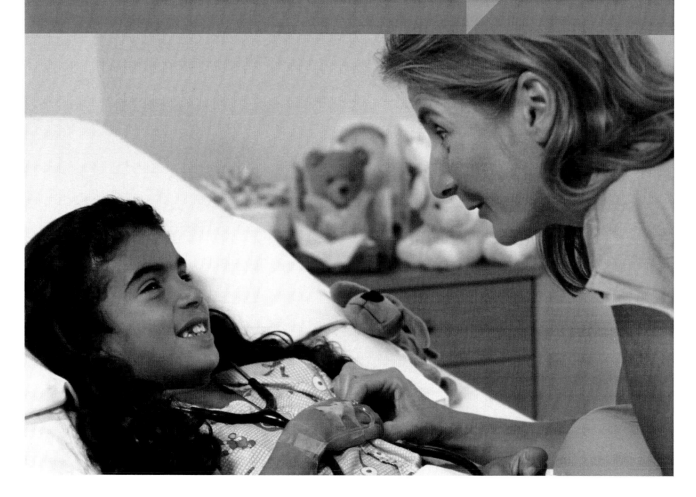

Authored by Andrea T. Cruz, M.D., M.P.H., F.A.A.P.,
*assistant professor of Pediatrics, Sections of Emergency Medicine
and Infectious Diseases, Baylor College of Medicine, Texas
Children's Hospital, and* **Coburn H. Allen, M.D., F.A.A.P.,**
*assistant professor of Pediatrics, Sections of Emergency
Medicine and Infectious Diseases, Baylor College
of Medicine, Texas Children's Hospital*

Infection control has been defined by the Centers for
Disease Control and Prevention (CDC) as the set of
guidelines that protect both patients and health care
workers from infectious diseases.[1] Infection control in these
settings is important, as nosocomial infections are major
causes of morbidity and mortality in adults and children,
contributing to approximately 99,000 estimated deaths
and 1.7 million infections in the United States in 2002.[2]
The mainstay for infection control is hand hygiene, with
frequent cleansing of the hands with either soap and water

or waterless antiseptic agents before and after patient contact. It is estimated that this inexpensive, low-technology strategy could prevent over half of nosocomial infections, as estimated by one study conducted in a neonatal intensive care unit.[3]

Most of the existing data on infection control practices are from the inpatient hospital setting, and there are few existing data on infection control as it relates to the emergency department (ED). There are several barriers to effective infection control in the ED, relative to other hospital settings. First, upon presentation to an ED, little to no laboratory data are often available to clinicians and other health care workers. Second, patients may not have yet presented with the full spectrum of symptomatology that might lead one to suspect a particular infectious etiology. Third, vital aspects of the history may be unavailable in the critically ill or mentally altered patient, particularly those who present to the ED unaccompanied by family or friends. Fourth, patients and families are often housed in close quarters in waiting rooms or multiple patient exam areas and have to share restrooms.

These same challenges also exist for pediatric patients and families presenting to EDs, and where a large percentage of visits are prompted by fever or other symptoms compatible with infectious diseases. The epidemiology of nosocomial infections in children is affected by (for the young child) immature immunological responses, lack of immunity via infection or passively by vaccination, closer contact between children and health care workers than seen in comparable adult settings, the role of toys as fomites, and the potential for siblings and adult family members to act as vectors of disease.[4] As many children utilize EDs as a primary care setting for acute illnesses, EDs have taken a more central role in disease surveillance. In the last decade, the theoretical and actual threats of bioterrorism and pandemic influenza have lent more importance to the role of surveillance in non-traditional settings. Given these challenges, the emphasis upon a systematic approach to infection control takes on even more importance in an ED setting.

This chapter will review the general principles of infection control as they relate to specific pathogens, symptoms, and procedures. The role of the ED in terms of surveillance for and response to bioterrorism and pandemic influenza will be discussed. Finally, commonly encountered scenarios will be reviewed. These include post-exposure prophylaxis, the evaluation of the child with a history of multidrug-resistant pathogens, isolation of the child or caregiver with suspected

tuberculosis, when health care workers should be held out of work, and post-exposure prophylaxis for patients and health care workers.

General Principles of Infection Control
Isolation Precautions

Isolation precautions relate to the child who is ill, in contrast with quarantine, a term used to describe the physical isolation of asymptomatic individuals potentially exposed to an infectious agent. Isolation precautions are generally classified as either standard or transmission-based.

Standard (Universal) Precautions

The spread of human immunodeficiency virus (HIV) led to the advent of standard (universal) precautions, wherein all patients are presumed to have blood-borne pathogens. These precautions are to be used with exposure to blood and all bodily secretions (with the exception of sweat), mucous membranes, and non-intact skin.[5] The components of standard precautions include the following items of personal protective equipment (PPE): hand hygiene, gloves, masks, impermeable gowns, face shields, and eye protection.

Hand hygiene should be universally used before and after contact with the patient. The ideal medium for hand hygiene is a waterless alcohol-based product, as these solutions are easy to use, have rapid onset of action, and offer a wide spectrum of antimicrobial activity.[1] The limitations to utility are ease of access (such as an empty canister of solution), the potential for skin desiccation after repeated utilizations, and discomfort if used over abraded skin. Alcohol-based solutions also lack a post-antimicrobial effect. The use of waterless products can replace soap and water in most settings, except in circumstances where there is visible soilage on the hands, at which point, soap and water should be used. In the ED setting, easy access to alcohol-based solutions for parents and children could also decrease transmission.

There are few pathogens that can survive the effects of alcohol- or detergent-based cleaning. For instance, *Clostridium difficile* can be resistant to alcohol-based cleansers, and mechanical scrubbing may be needed to remove spores from hands. Additionally, bleach-containing disinfectants can be used for *C. difficile*.[6] Norovirus is another pathogen that is relatively resistant to routine disinfection. One nosocomial outbreak was only terminated with closure of several hospital units and disinfection with sodium hypochlorite, at a total cost of over half a million dollars.[7] The use of gloves does not obviate the need for

TABLE 5-1

Transmission-Based Precautions for Specific Infectious Diseases

Precaution	Equipment*	Pathogens
Contact	Gown; gloves	Multidrug-resistant bacteria§, anthrax (cutaneous), *Brucella* (if draining wound), cholera (if incontinent), *Clostridium difficile*, conjunctivitis, diarrheal disease (if incontinent), diphtheria (cutaneous), enteroviruses, *E. coli* O157:H7, hemorrhagic fever viruses, hepatitis A, herpes simplex virus, herpes zoster, impetigo, lice, parainfluenza virus, respiratory syncytial virus, rotavirus, severe acute respiratory syndrome (SARS)[†], scabies, *Shigella* skin/soft tissue infections, smallpox, *Staphylococcus aureus* (cutaneous), and viral hemorrhagic fevers
Airborne	Private, negative-pressure room; fitted N95 respirator for health care workers	Tuberculosis, measles, varicella, SARS[†], smallpox
Droplet	Private room (if possible); mask if within three feet of patient	Adenovirus, diphtheria (pharyngeal), *Haemophilus influenza* type B, hemorrhagic fever viruses, influenza, mumps, *Mycoplasma pneumoniae*, *Neisseria meningitidis*, parvovirus B19, pertussis, plague (pneumonic), rubella, SARS[†], group A streptococcus

* Hand hygiene should be used before and after all patient contact, regardless of the suspected or proven pathogen.
[†] Some experts recommend the use of contact, droplet, and airborne precautions for SARS.
§ Multidrug-resistant organisms are defined by CDC as organisms resistant to at least one class of antimicrobials.

Adapted from Siegel J.D., Rhinehart E., Jackson M., Chairello L., and the Healthcare Infection Control Practices Advisory Committee: 2007 Guideline for isolation precautions: preventing transmission of infectious agents in healthcare settings. June 2007. http://www.cdc.gov/ncidod/dhqp/pdf/isolation2007.pdf.

American Academy of Pediatrics. Pickering L.K. (ed.): *2006 Red Book: Report of the Committee on Infectious Diseases.* 27th ed. Elk Grove Village, IL: American Academy of Pediatrics, 2006.

hand hygiene. The use of other components of PPE is dependent on the procedure being performed, as will be discussed in a later section.

Transmission-based Precautions

These precautions are supplemental measures taken to protect health care workers and other patients from pathogens requiring additional barriers. Such measures are based in part on the size of aerosolized particles, the dispersal of particles in indoor settings, the ability of particles to remain airborne for long periods, and the viability of the pathogen on non-biologic surfaces. Transmission-based precautions are subdivided into three groups: contact, airborne, and droplet precautions. The pathogens in each category, as well as the PPE and facilities necessary, are listed in Table 5-1, above.

The most important route of transmission for nosocomial infections is via contact transmission, whereby there is physical acquisition and transfer of microbes either directly from a patient or indirectly via a fomite or through the contaminated hands of health care workers. Many of the pathogens transmitted in this manner can be viable outside the body for long periods of time, are resistant to routinely utilized cleansers, or both.

There are few common pathogens requiring airborne-transmission precautions: tuberculosis, measles, and varicella (SARS and smallpox also require airborne precautions). These infections are characterized by wide and prolonged pathogen dispersal in indoor settings due to small particle size, necessitating negative-pressure rooms and NIOSH-certified, fit-tested respirators (N95 face masks).

Droplet transmission can be either direct or indirect from exposure to particles aerosolized for brief periods. In contrast to airborne transmission, pathogen-laden particles are heavier, therefore traveling shorter distances (three feet or less), and tend not to remain aerosolized for long periods. These pathogens do not require special ventilation systems such as negative-pressure rooms. However, facial protection is necessary given the risk of droplets contacting mucosal surfaces.

Specific Symptoms

Transmission-based precautions should be quickly implemented based on the patient's symptoms, not on the results of diagnostic testing. Often, isolation precautions are only implemented *after* pathogen identification (e.g., rotavirus assay is positive). However, rapid diagnostic assays are not infallible, nor do we have tests for all the potential causes of likely infectious disorders such as diarrheal disease or upper respiratory tract infections. Consequently, transmission precautions should be begun empirically. The examples of bronchiolitis, diarrheal disease, and skin and soft tissue infections are reviewed. The management of a health care worker with similar infections is described in a later section.

Bronchiolitis, caused by respiratory syncytial virus (RSV), parainfluenza viruses, and other viral pathogens or organisms, causes significant morbidity each year, with RSV alone accounting for more than 90,000 hospitalizations annually. There is substantial variation in the onset and duration of the RSV season geographically, with longer seasons seen in more southern states.[8] It is estimated that up to 40% of nosocomial RSV infections in young infants are associated with lower respiratory tract disease,[9] with particularly severe consequences in neonatal intensive care and hematology/ oncology units. Strategies that have worked in these settings to decrease nosocomial transmission include cohorting of nurses and patients, compliance with handwashing techniques, and (occasionally) use of palivizumab, the monoclonal RSV antibody, to limit spread.[10] However, the feasibility of many of these strategies in the ED setting is questionable. The American Academy of Pediatrics stresses several points regarding efforts to prevent nosocomial spread of the viruses causing bronchiolitis. These include emphasizing the role of hand hygiene, preferably with alcohol-based products, in preventing nosocomial transmission; use of gowns and gloves for direct patient contact; educating families about preventing spread; early triage of ED pediatric patients with upper and lower respiratory

symptoms into an exam room and away from a crowded waiting area; and implementing RSV surveillance early in the season.[11] Contact precautions should be utilized in all patients with clinical bronchiolitis, not solely in those with a positive RSV test.

One frequently encountered ED presentation is the child with diarrhea. It is estimated that there are up to 35 million episodes of diarrheal disease annually in children under five years of age in the United States. Despite the recent introduction of the rotavirus vaccine, this remains a common complaint among children and their caregivers. One recent study showed that while the rates of inpatient admissions for diarrhea have been stable in the last decade, ED visits for diarrhea have doubled over that interval.[12] Pathogens are identified in a minority of cases, but the most commonly isolated organisms include adenovirus, rotavirus, astrovirus, and norovirus.[13] Bacterial pathogens are uncommon causes of acute, nonbloody diarrhea in the child lacking a travel history. The only cause of diarrheal disease for which a rapid test exists is rotavirus, which accounts for 5%–50% of all cases.[14] Thus, children with diarrhea who are incontinent or still in diapers should be placed on contact (barrier) precautions from the initial evaluation.[4]

Skin and soft tissue infections (SSTIs) have been increasing in frequency in the last decade. The primary causes are *Staphylococcus aureus* and group A streptococcus. Methicillin-resistant *S. aureus* (MRSA) has also increased in frequency, with MRSA accounting for almost 80% of staphylococcal isolates in some areas.[15] The CDC recommends contact precautions for major draining abscesses until the drainage stops or it can be contained by a dressing,[4] as well as for children with MRSA infections. However, at the time a child is seen in the ED for an SSTI, drug susceptibilities are usually not available. Consequently, empiric contact precautions should be utilized for all children with draining wounds.

Specific Procedures

Guidelines exist regarding the usage of PPE for specific procedures. These guidelines are based on anticipated risk of exposure and the type of isolation the patient is already on. For instance, if there is concern about blood splash from a procedure, a mask, eye/face shield, and impermeable gown should be selected for PPE. In general, it would be prudent to anticipate the most significant exposure from a given procedure and plan accordingly. The PPE recommendations for some common ED procedures are listed in Table 5-2, page 79.

TABLE 5-2

Procedure-Specific Guidelines for the Use of Personal Protective Equipment (PPE)

Procedure	Gloves	Gown	Mask	Eye/face shield	Hair covering
Intubation	+		+	+	
Suctioning	+		+	+	
Central line placement	+	+	+	+	+
Chest tube placement	+	+	+	+	+
CPR	+		+	+	
Incision and drainage of abscess	+		+	+	
Wound repairs	+				

Adapted from Centers for Disease Control and Prevention. Personal protective equipment (PPE) in healthcare settings. http://www.cdc.gov/ncidod/dhqp/ppe.html (accessed Aug. 30, 2008).

PPE should be donned prior to patient contact and after hand hygiene. After the procedure or evaluation is completed, equipment should be discarded in specified receptacles and hand hygiene again implemented. Although the particular combination of PPE will influence the order in which equipment is donned, in general the gown is placed first, followed by the mask, eye or face shield, and finally gloves. The proper order for removing PPE should be followed to minimize risk of self-contamination: first, gloves are removed, followed by eye/face shield, gown, and mask.[16]

Vaccines Recommended for Health Care Workers

Most vaccines recommended for health care workers are also recommended for the general adult populace (see Table 5-3 on page 80). An exception is the meningococcal vaccine, which is recommended for microbiologists in routine contact with *Neisseria menigitidis,* as well as for adolescents, but is not currently recommended for health care workers. It is now recommended that the traditional Td booster for tetanus be replaced with the TDaP, as adults with waning immunity to pertussis often are the source of severe disease in young children in the community.[17] From the

perspective of health care workers, receipt of the TDaP vaccine does not preclude the need for antibiotic prophylaxis in the event of a pertussis exposure, as vaccination is only 75% to 85% protective.[18]

Surveillance

The historic function of EDs has been the management of acute illnesses; however, the notion that the ED might also play a vital role in surveillance for infectious diseases might not seem obvious. This section will review several basic practices and models of surveillance that are natural to the ED setting, including the basic models that may be used for infectious disease surveillance; existing networks; and reportable diseases. Finally, the example of severe acute respiratory syndrome (SARS) will be utilized to link the concept of surveillance to bioterrorism and pandemic influenza.

The ED is a logical location in which to conduct disease surveillance for many reasons. First, the ED serves as the primary care provider to millions of uninsured and underinsured Americans. Many of these individuals are at relatively higher risk for certain infections than the general

TABLE 5-3

Vaccines Recommended for Health Care Workers

Vaccine*	# Doses	Schedule	Other
Hepatitis B	3	0,1,6 months	Serologies should be obtained after last vaccine in series to confirm immunologic response.
Influenza	1	Annual	Can be administered intramuscularly (IM) or intranasally; the inactivated IM vaccine is recommended for health care workers in close contact with severely immunocompromised patients.
Measles, mumps, rubella	2	0,4 weeks	For healh care workers born after 1956 without serologic evidence of immunity.
Meningococcal	1	Once	Recommended only for microbiologists exposed to the organism in the laboratory setting; not recommended *a priori* for ED staff and health care workers.
Tetanus, Diphtheria, Pertussis	1	10-year booster	TDaP should replace Td boosters for all adults. Health care workers can be immunized with TDaP as soon as two years after receipt of the last Td booster.
Varicella	2	0,4 weeks	For health care workers without serologic evidence of immunity, history of varicella, or documentation of immunization.

* Contraindications to vaccination based on egg or other allergies or immune status should be reviewed by the health care worker and employee health practitioner prior to all immunizations.

Adapted from Centers for Disease Control and Prevention. *Vaccinations for healthcare workers.* http://www.cdc.gov/vaccines/spec-grps/hcw.htm (accessed Aug. 30, 2008).

populace, and disease in marginalized populations can be a harbinger of the same disease in other sectors of the population. Second, the diagnostic capabilities of most hospitals exceed that of most community health care providers. Certain laboratory tests might be more readily available or have a faster turn-around time in hospital settings. Third, the sheer number of patients seen in many EDs might make pattern recognition easier for many infectious diseases. In a local clinic with lower patient flow volumes, increases in numbers of disease syndromes might not be as readily apparent. Fourth, these data can be real-time, in contrast to traditional passive methods of disease surveillance, where gaps of up to two weeks between symptom onset and disease recognition are common. Data from the ED can be analyzed prospectively through the electronic medical record (EMR) or immediately from a retrospective view if desired. Fifth, these are data (demographic, chief complaint) that are already being collected, minimizing the burden on an already overtaxed system. Finally, surveillance data have the chance to impact

the care of patients. For example, knowing that influenza is already being seen in a given community could serve as an impetus to increase immunization rates and to test for and treat at-risk children with influenza-like illnesses who might benefit from early antiviral therapy.[19]

At least three different systems have been used to conduct surveillance in EDs and other acute-care settings. These include EMERGEncy ID NET, Real-time Outbreak and Disease Surveillance (RODS), and the Bio-Surveillance Analysis, Feedback, Evaluation, and Response (B-SAFER) system.[20, 21, 22] These systems use a variety of data points, including triage chief complaints, discharge diagnoses, prescriptions written, and laboratory results as adjunctive measures to increase traditional public health surveillance. In particular, symptom- or syndrome-based surveillance patterns have been able to be identified early into the evolution of an epidemic.[22] One of the commonalities of these different systems is that all are based upon data elements already being gathered by clinicians. The ability to rapidly abstract these data from electronic medical records offers the potential for real-time surveillance and early recognition of disease patterns that lie outside the spectrum of what is normally seen by regional EDs. Another way to conduct ED surveillance is based on patient/family response to questionnaires. For example, with burgeoning concerns about swine and avian influenza, some facilities screened families by asking about contact with swine or poultry. Many pediatric EDs ask questions about exposure to individuals with varicella, recognizing the ease of spread of this virus and the implications for immunocompromised patients.

There are limitations to surveillance in the ED. The main limitation is that, in order to recognize deviations in expected patterns of symptoms or diagnoses, it is necessary to first establish a baseline for what is considered the norm. In the ED, variations in disease patterns may be due to daily variations in patient volume (for example, most EDs find Monday to be the busiest day of the week) or to variations in clinical presentation that are extrinsic to the disease itself and that are more rooted in socioeconomic concerns (such as availability of providers outside the ED). Another limitation is that the role of surveillance is typically one that has been outside the purview of the ED clinician. Education on the utility of surveillance to the care of the individual patient needs to be emphasized in order to obtain cooperation on the part of ED staff, as infection control is not something that may have been emphasized in the formal training curriculum for many ED care providers.

The list of reportable infectious diseases may vary slightly by state. However, the CDC has compiled a list of diseases that require notification across the country. The time frame for reporting does vary by disease, depending in part on disease severity, potential for use as an agent of bioterrorism, and level of infectivity. This annually updated list is available online at www.cdc.gov/epo/dphsi/phs/infdis.htm.[23] In many hospitals, notification of the local or state health department falls under the purview of the clinical laboratory in the case of positive cultures or serologic assays. In the ED setting, the results of diagnostic assays are often unavailable at the time a child is being seen. However, prompt reporting increases the passive surveillance capabilities of the current system. ED clinical leadership should partner with hospital laboratory and infection control departments to assure that there is a system in place for the systematic review of pertinent positive and negative cultures and serologic tests obtained in the ED, with processes for notification of the patient, the patient's medical home, and, when indicated, the local or state health department.

In 2003, reports out of Hong Kong and Toronto described an outbreak of a severe illness that caused respiratory collapse and death in previously healthy adults. Severe acute respiratory syndrome (SARS), caused by a novel coronavirus, was rapidly identified and infection control measures limited its spread both within and outside the hospital. The example of SARS served as a sentinel event for infection control practitioners already concerned about the specter of bioterrorism and pandemic influenza, and many of the lessons from SARS are applicable to both domains. The CDC, in combination with health care providers from Toronto facilities, where transmission within hospital settings contributed heavily to disease burden, pointed out five lessons to be learned from SARS, applicable both to future SARS outbreaks and, more broadly, to other respiratory pathogens.[24] These lessons include:

1. A coordinated response by multiple groups was needed.

2. Unrecognized, presumably milder, cases of SARS served as significant sources of in-hospital transmission.

3. Restricting access to hospitals, both by diverting patients and redirecting workload on existing health care workers, served to minimize transmission.

4. While airborne (and contact and droplet) precautions were recommended, several barriers (e.g., patient volume leading to lack of negative-pressure rooms; hospital overcrowding) made these precautions impossible to implement in all cases.

5. Transmission of SARS to staff and the policy of quarantining health care workers exposed to infection led to staffing shortages.

All these lessons are applicable to the threats of bioterrorism and pandemic influenza. Although we might still be caught without all needed resources, adequate biosurveillance can result in a greater lead-time to divert resources, determine alternative isolation facilities, and increase health care worker staffing.

Bioterrorism

In the wake of September 11th and the anthrax attacks, there has been increasing concern about the use of biological agents as weapons of terror. The infections that fall into this category share several features. First, the population would be highly susceptible. Second, these pathogens cause significant morbidity and mortality. Third, they are relatively easy to manufacture and disperse. Fourth, for some agents, there is the possibility of secondary transmission within the community. Fifth, there are limited diagnostic and therapeutic options widely available for

TABLE 5-4			

Infections Agents Considered to Be Bioterrorist Threats and Pathogen-specific Isolation Precautions

Category	Ease of Dissemination	Morbidity/ Mortality	Agents
A	++	++	Anthrax,[1] botulism, plague,[3] smallpox,[1,2] tularemia, viral hemorrhagic fevers[1,3]
B	+	+	*Brucella,*[1] *Clostridum perfringens,* food safety threats (Gram-negative enterics),[1] glanders, melioidosis, Q fever, staphylococcal enterotoxin B,[1] typhus, viral encephalitis viruses, water safety threats *(Vibrio, Cryptosporidium)*[1]
C	– (currently)	++	Hantavirus, Nipah virus

Isolation precautions: [1]contact; [2]airborne; [3]droplet. The remaining agents require standard precautions.

Adapted from Centers for Disease Control and Prevention. http://www.bt.cdc.gov/agent/agentlist (accessed Sep.1, 2008).

many of these pathogens. Finally, all these pathogens have the ability to cause significant psychological distress to the affected population(s).[25]

The CDC list of bioterrorism threats are categorized according to ease of dissemination, morbidity, and mortality in a susceptible population, and available diagnostic (and surveillance) tools. The most imminent threats are Category A agents, whereas Category C agents are emerging infections that have potential as bioterrorism threats in the future but not at present (see Table 5-4, above).

Following the SARS outbreak in surrounding countries in southeast Asia, a hospital in Singapore reported its experiences with SARS surveillance and infection control in their ED. They used SARS as a model for bioterrorism attacks and noted some ED-specific interventions that might be applicable in other circumstances.[27] First, a screening questionnaire was used to elicit a history of travel and specific symptoms; this was used to stratify patients as low-, medium-, or high-risk. Second, at-risk patients were issued surgical masks. Third, an adjacent facility (previously used for decontamination) was used to triage and evaluate high-risk patients, thus bypassing the main ED. Fourth, patients were placed outdoors under tents while waiting for evaluation and during triage. Fifth, staff were restricted to working with patients in certain areas, to minimize potential cross-

infection. Sixth, visitations were restricted (which would clearly be more difficult to accomplish in pediatric settings, where parents often provide care that would otherwise be accomplished by nursing staff). Finally, there was prompt reporting to public health authorities and real-time surveillance of computerized triage logs. Together, this system identified the majority of patients with SARS, almost all patients who did not have SARS, and eliminated spread from patients to staff or to other patients in the ED at the same time. Many of these measures could be implemented in most EDs in the United States.

EDs can prepare for a bioterrorism event in several ways. First, clinicians and other health care workers can be educated on the symptoms and precautions needed for the Category A agents. One study looked at using interactive screen savers with rotating textual and graphical information on potential bioterrorism agents. This was coupled with web-based resources that could be easily accessed and downloaded from all hospital computers,[28] resulting in a 30% increase in health care worker knowledge of bioterrorism agents. Second, surveillance systems, especially those that are syndrome- or symptom-based abstractions from an electronic medical record, can rapidly discern disease patterns early in an outbreak. Third, hospitals should have specific guidelines regarding isolation and reporting. Finally, hospitals should identify alternative resources, both physical and human, that may be utilized in the event of bioterrorism or a mass casualty event.[25, 27]

Once a patient with a potential infection from a bioterrorism agent presents to the ED, transmission precautions should be immediately implemented, and early communication with infection control practitioners, infectious disease specialists, and regional health departments should begin immediately. An algorithm for this process was created by Ollerton,[25] and is presented in Figure 5-1 on page 84.

Although a detailed overview of the bioterrorism agents is outside the scope of this chapter, Table 5-5, page 87, briefly discusses the general symptoms, isolation precautions, post-exposure prophylaxis, and vaccines (when applicable) for Category A bioterrorism agents. Excellent reviews of the clinical presentation, epidemiology, diagnosis, and treatment of these pathogens, from both the pediatric and ED perspectives are available.[29, 30]

In summary, given the lack of a personal knowledge base about these pathogens, the fact that many may mimic routine pathogens or initially present with nonspecific symptoms, and the high degree of infectivity associated with these infections, an active surveillance system, a high index of suspicion, and pre-existing infection control protocols will be needed to recognize and control these threats.

Pandemic Influenza

In the last decade, increased transmission of avian influenza has been noted in Southeast Asia and other countries. To date, there have been few cases of effective human-to-human transmission of avian influenza; once this occurs, pandemic influenza is seemingly inevitable. Pandemic influenza, as demonstrated recently by the H1N1 pandemic, poses several challenges to ED practitioners. These include increased resource utilization; staffing concerns; diagnostic and treatment difficulties; and the lack of known effective preventive strategies. Resource utilization includes all of the following: total ED visits and ED visits for patients with severe respiratory distress and failure; the need to stockpile antiviral therapies; the need for adequate PPE for health care workers; and sufficient ventilators for critically ill patients. Staffing concerns surround health care worker absenteeism because of nosocomially transmitted influenza, care for affected health care worker family members (especially children), and the fear of acquiring a potentially deadly virus in the workplace. The experience with SARS suggested that cohorting staff with infected

patients is effective; however, the logistics of implementing this in the ED setting are unclear. Diagnostic and therapeutic concerns also abound. Currently available rapid diagnostic tests for influenza virus types A and B (seasonal epidemics) show suboptimal sensitivity. It is unclear how well these assays would perform for recombinant viruses capable of pandemic disease. Therapeutic issues include that there are limited data on the efficacy of currently available antivirals in the treatment of avian or pandemic influenza. For conventional influenza viruses approximately 20% of isolates are resistant to antivirals by the time a seven-day treatment course is completed.[31] The efficacy of prevention strategies, using the same agents (oseltamivir, zanamivir) used to treat influenza virus, is unknown, and the prolonged period during which antiviral chemoprophylaxis would be necessary means that current antiviral stockpiles would be inadequate to cover the United States population. While the H1N1 virus appears to remain sensitive to the agents (as of late fall 2009), concerns also remain regarding the development of resistance with excessive use of antiviral drugs.

Most plans for pandemic influenza preparedness have included at least six tenets. First, improvements are needed in diagnostic virology capabilities and surveillance systems. Second, vaccinations should be prioritized depending on vaccine supply. Third, barriers to vaccine development (inadequate funding for research and liability protection) need to be addressed. Fourth, novel antiviral agents and increasing the supply of existing antivirals is necessary. Fifth, local and national communications need to be in place to allow rapid information dissemination to other clinicians and patients. Finally, community-based preparedness plans need to be well thought out prior to the advent of pandemic influenza.[32]

Several measures for infection control and surveillance can be accomplished in the ED. First, screening questionnaires asking about travel history and poultry contact have worked well in many countries in Southeast Asia. Second, respiratory and hand hygiene and cough etiquette will be important in decreasing nosocomial transmission. Droplet precautions are indicated for patients with suspected influenza (seasonal or pandemic). These measures should be implemented in any patient with an influenza-like illness. One study of health care worker adherence with respiratory infection control practices showed that, while awareness and knowledge were adequate, adherence with recommendations remained poor, especially for hand hygiene after touching equipment in patient rooms and the use of gloves and

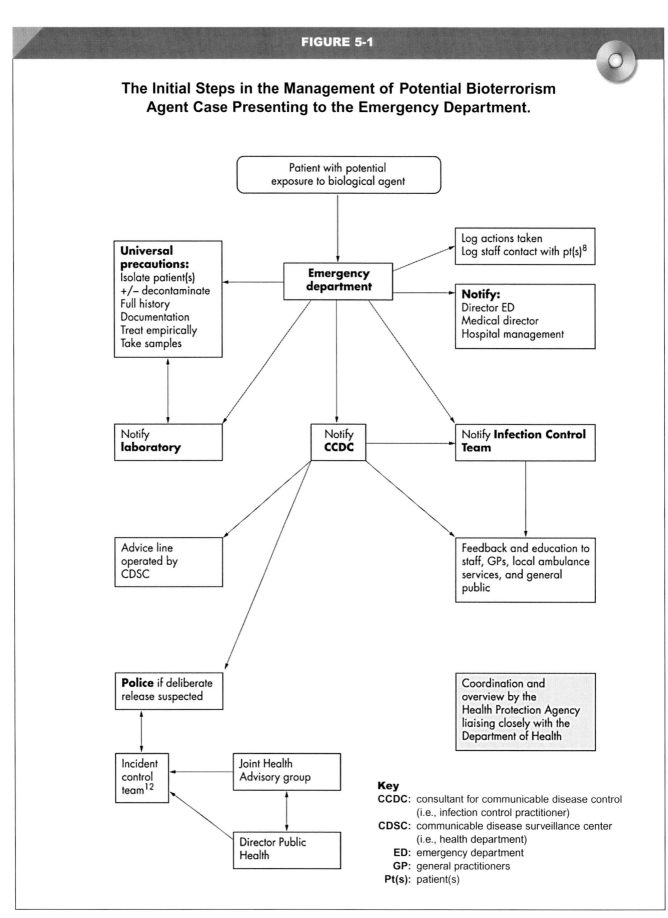

FIGURE 5-1

The Initial Steps in the Management of Potential Bioterrorism Agent Case Presenting to the Emergency Department.

Reproduced from Ollerton J.E.: Emergency department response to the deliberate release of biological agents. *Emerg Med J* 21:5–8, 2004 with permission from BMJ Publishing Group, Ltd.

masks.[33] Third, a case definition is necessary to enable more accurate screening for influenza disease. This definition should be in a format that could easily be imported into existing triage protocols and electronic medical record systems to allow more accurate surveillance. Fourth, immunization with conventional influenza should continue to be recommended for all health care workers, as immunization would decrease the possibility that an individual could harbor both conventional and pandemic influenza, thereby decreasing possibilities for genetic reassortment and might offer potential cross-protection.

One simulation study in an ED and inpatient unit modeled the impact of pandemic influenza.[34] In this study, there was variable compliance among health care workers with PPE: each patient required up to 25 sets of PPE and had contact with a mean of 12 health care workers, and up to 41% of health care workers, close contacts would have qualified for antiviral post-exposure prophylaxis. Environmental decontamination was suboptimal. These data indicate that existing supplies of antiviral therapies and PPE are insufficient. Most post-exposure prophylaxis was needed in ED health care workers, where the diagnosis was often not immediately suspected and isolation procedures were not immediately implemented. Thus, the importance of ED-based, rapid, practical infection control practices is as important with pandemic influenza as it is for other pathogens.

The recent ED experience with H1N1 swine influenza in 2009 reinforced many of these messages. At Texas Children's Hospital, patients were triaged out of doors and well-appearing children with influenza-like illnesses received all their care in an open-air region outside of the main ED. The goal here was to minimize egress into the building for non-urgent visits by children and guardians with respiratory infections, to promote early patient cohorting by symptoms in separate waiting areas, and to increase respiratory etiquette through the use of face masks and hand sanitizers. Implementation of this mobile pediatric emergency response team led to decreased waiting times for all children in the ED (despite up to 50% increases in patient volume over seasonal baselines), fewer children who left prior to medical evaluation, and enabled the ED to mobilize existing institutional resources and infrastructure to deal with a new pathogen.

Specific Infection Control Scenarios

A number of situations with infection control implications occur on a regular basis in many EDs. These include the child with a history of drug-resistant infections, the

chronically ill child, the isolation precautions needed for children with suspected tuberculosis, post-exposure prophylaxis for patients (and their relatives) and health care workers, when to hold health care workers out of work, and the management of the under-immunized health care worker in outbreak situations.

Multidrug-Resistant Organisms

Multidrug-resistant organisms (MDROs) are usually defined as bacteria not susceptible to at least one class of antibiotics.[35] MDROs are transmitted in the same manner as their drug-susceptible counterparts. However, the consequences of nosocomial transmission are more severe. The most frequently encountered pathogens are MRSA, vancomycin-resistant enterococci (VRE), MDR-*Pseudomonas aeruginosa* (particularly in the cystic fibrosis population), and Gram-negative bacilli producing extended spectrum beta-lactamases (ESBL). In the pediatric population, the latter have primarily included *E. coli* and *Klebsiella* species. More recently, invasive infections with MDR-pneumococcal isolates (serotype 19A) have been reported.[36]

Most of these MDROs are transmitted by direct contact, or in the case of cystic fibrosis patients, in congregate settings both within and outside the hospital.[37] Strict use of barrier precautions, patient isolation, surveillance cultures, communicating laboratory results of prior admissions to admitting clinicians, and flagging the charts of patients with MDROs[38] have been used in the past with various levels of success. However, implementation of these measures across institutions has not been systematic, and the efficacy of these interventions is unclear.[39] In the ED setting, rapid identification and use of barrier precautions in children with a history of MDROs could limit nosocomial spread of infections. As more facilities move toward electronic medical records, color-coded and textual prompts could be utilized to inform personnel of patients with these histories.

The Chronically Ill Child

The child with chronic illness poses special infection control challenges. These children often have had extensive contact with the health care system and prolonged or frequent antibiotic exposure. As such, they are at risk for MDROs, as described in the previous section. The prevalence of vancomycin-resistant enterococci (VRE) in hemodialysis patients and the multidrug-resistant *Burkholderia* and *Pseudomonas* species seen in cystic fibrosis patients, as well as the role of the inpatient setting in facilitating transmission, have been well described.[40] However, children who might not be generally classified as chronically ill, but who nonetheless have had repetitive antibiotic exposure can also have ESBL-producing species of *E. coli* and *Klebsiella*.[41] Review of culture data from prior encounters can facilitate decision-making about isolation in the ED setting.

The chronically ill child also poses challenges because some are technologically dependent with devices that require special care and precautions in acute care settings and might also serve as portals of entry for infectious pathogens. The best example in the ED is the child with a tracheostomy with increased secretions. Suctioning and obtaining of cultures in these patients should be undertaken using the precautions outlined in Table 5-2, page 79. Finally, many neurologically impaired children are incontinent well into childhood and adolescence, requiring contact precautions in many circumstances.

The Child with Suspected Tuberculosis

A child being evaluated in the ED for suspected pulmonary tuberculosis (TB) should be placed in a negative-pressure room. Health care workers entering the room should wear N95 fit-tested respirators. When the child is transported outside the room, the patient and caregivers should wear standard surgical masks. As non-employees have not been fit-tested, N95 respirators should not be used for these individuals. Routine surgical masks serve to decrease aerosolization. In facilities without negative-pressure rooms, patients should wear surgical masks and change them when wet.[42] Tuberculosis is relatively resistant to standard germicidal cleansers, and requires disinfection with intermediate level cleaners.[43] Decontamination with hydrogen peroxide vapor has also been effectively utilized in small enclosed spaces.[44]

One facet of infection control related to TB in children is that the pre-pubertal child is infrequently contagious. However, any child with acid-fast bacilli (AFB)-positive sputum smears, extensive pulmonary infiltrates, cavitary disease, laryngeal disease, or an infant with suspected congenital TB should be treated as contagious.[5] A child (or adult) with a positive tuberculin skin test (PPD) and a normal chest radiograph does not require isolation.

In the pediatric population, the greatest risk is not from the patient, but from the caregiver who accompanies the child to the ED. One study conducted in an area of relatively high TB prevalence in the United States showed that in more than 15% of children with suspected TB, the person who accompanied them to the ED was the person from whom the child acquired infection. Consequently, this can influence hospital policy, for instance, by mandating chest radiographs (at hospital expense) for parents/caregivers of children with suspected TB.[45] The adults are kept either in the room without masks or outside the room with surgical masks until the chest radiograph have been interpreted. This policy has the potential to greatly decrease spread of the organism in hospital settings. Prolonged wait times, overcrowded waiting rooms, and a paucity of negative-pressure isolation rooms all contribute to the difficulties with implementing TB-appropriate precautions in the ED.[46]

Post-Exposure Prophylaxis

Post-exposure prophylaxis (PEP) is not an infrequent reason for presentation to the pediatric ED, especially in cases where community-based resources are limited. This section is subdivided into discussions of PEP for patients and their families and PEP for health care workers. The former section covers the management of the child and family exposed to various infectious agents (measles, meningococcus, mumps, pertussis, rabies), and a general approach to a child potentially exposed to blood-borne pathogens. PEP for health care workers will focus upon needlestick injuries and exposure to other blood-borne pathogens and occupational exposures to meningitis and pertussis. PEP for agents of bioterrorism are described within that section.

Patients and Families

In the ED, PEP for pediatric patients or families typically falls into a few discrete circumstances: the child or family exposed to pertussis, measles, mumps, or meningococcal meningitis; the child with animal exposure and concern for rabies; and evaluation of the child who has potentially been exposed to blood-borne pathogens. In these circumstances, quantifying the risk can be difficult given often unavailable immunization records and different perspectives on the amount of exposure a patient had to an animal or another individual.

Pertussis is a re-emerging disease nationwide, in part because of waning immunity in adolescents and young adults, which prompted the 2005 recommendation that tetanus boosters also contain the acellular pertussis vaccine component (TDaP) when adults are re-boosted. Infants < 6 months, particularly Hispanic infants, bear most of the disease burden in terms of morbidity and mortality. When a child is evaluated for suspected pertussis, several things must occur. First, the child should immediately be placed in droplet isolation (for example, isolation should *precede*, not *follow*, microbiologic confirmation). Second, underimmunized children less than seven years of age

TABLE 5-5

Common Symptoms, Isolation Precautions, and Post-Exposure Interventions for Category A Bioterrorism Agents for Asymptomatic Persons

Disease	Symptoms	Isolation precautions	Post-exposure prophylaxis	Vaccine availability	Decontamination
Anthrax	Eschar (cutaneous); respiratory distress, widened mediastinum (inhalational)	Standard; if have draining eschar, use contact precautions	Ciprofloxacin or doxycycline (antibiotics should be given for 60 days)	Yes, for high-risk individuals; not adequate for PEP	Sodium hypochlorite; gamma radiation
Botulism	Descending paralysis; diplopia; dysphagia; dysarthria; dysphonia	Standard	Antitoxin not routinely recommended because of scarcity and high rates of hypersensitivity reactions	Investigational vaccine available for laboratory workers alone; not effective for PEP	Sodium hypochlorite
Hemorrhagic fever viruses	Fever; petechiae; bleeding	Droplet, Contact	Supportive; ribavirin has some efficacy in disease, but not in PEP	None	Standard
Plague	Fever; pneumonia; tender lympha-denopathy	Standard; if pneumonic plague, use droplet precautions	Doxycycline, trimethoprim-sulfamethoxazole, or ciprofloxacin (antibiotics should be given for 7 days)	None available in the U.S. Prior vaccine ineffective against pneumonic plague	Standard
Smallpox	Fever; vesicular centrifugal rash	Standard, contact, airborne	Supportive. Cidofovir may be useful for PEP, but is investigational and has significant nephrotoxicity	Yes (within 4 days); Vaccinia immune globulin for immuno-compromised individuals or others who cannot tolerate vaccination	Standard agents, but thorough cleansing (virus can persist up to 24 hours after release)
Tularemia	Fever; pneumonia	Standard (no human-to-human transmission)	Ciprofloxacin or doxycycline (antibiotics should be given for 14 days) if have bioterrorism or environmental exposure	Available for laboratory workers; no efficacy for PEP	Standard

PEP: post-exposure prophylaxis

Adapted from American Academy of Pediatrics. Pickering L.K., (ed.): *2006 Red Book: Report of the Committee on Infectious Diseases.* 27th ed. Elk Grove Village, IL: American Academy of Pediatrics; 2006.

Patt H.A., Feigin R.D.: Diagnosis and management of suspected cases of bioterrorism: a pediatric perspective. *Pediatrics* 109:685–692, 2002.

Kman N.E., Nelson R.N.: Infectious agents of bioterrorism: a review for emergency physicians. *Emerg Med Clin N Am* 26:517–547, 2008.

should be vaccinated. Third, all household and other close contacts should be offered chemoprophylaxis, regardless of vaccination status or age, to limit secondary transmission.[5] The optimal therapeutic options are macrolide antibiotics such as azithromycin or clarithromycin; trimethoprim-sulfamethoxazole (twice daily for 14 days) can be used for patients with macrolide allergies. Although erythromycin can be used, the more frequent dosing interval (four times daily) and higher risk of gastrointestinal distress makes macrolides a more palatable option for most patients.

Measles and mumps are also re-emerging diseases, in part because levels of immunity need to be so high (greater than 90%) to offer herd immunity that underimmunized individuals are at high risk during times of community outbreaks. The MMR vaccine has been more effective PEP for measles than for mumps but remains recommended for both. The vaccine should be given within 72 hours of exposure, and the measles immune globulin should be administered within six days of exposure. Mumps immune globulin is not effective PEP and is no longer available in the United States. The guidelines for individuals for whom measles immunization is recommended are outlined in the Red Book.[5] Generally, measles immune globulin is recommended for immunocompromised or pregnant persons, infants under 12 months, and household or close contacts who are unimmunized.

The child with suspected bacterial meningitis should be treated with droplet precautions in the event that it is meningococcal meningitis. Although this can be more easily suspected in the child with meningismus and a purpuric rash, not infrequently the diagnosis is established after ED disposition. Close or household contact or persons in contact with respiratory secretions of patients with meningococcal meningitis should be offered prophylaxis. For children under 18 years of age, rifampin (twice daily for two days) or a single intramuscular dose of ceftriaxone is recommended. For adults, ciprofloxacin (500 mg single dose) is another alternative. Pregnant women exposed to meningococcus should receive ceftriaxone. All regimens are equally efficacious (90% to 95%). Optimally, PEP would begin within 24 hours of diagnosis in the source case; chemoprophylaxis has little documented benefit after 14 days of exposure.[5] The quadravalent conjugate meningococcal vaccine (Menactra®) can also be used in community-wide outbreaks, as the risk period can often extend for several weeks. At this point, it is still recommended that individuals who have received the meningococcal vaccine and are subsequently exposed also be offered

chemoprophylaxis. *Haemophilus influenzae* type B (Hib) meningitis is now uncommon but is sometimes seen in unimmunized children. In these instances, chemoprophylaxis is suggested for households with children under four years of age and incompletely immunized or households with immunocompromised children, regardless of immunization status.[5] The recommended agent is rifampin, which should be administered immediately after confirmation of Hib meningitis or other invasive disease; rifampin offers minimal benefit after seven days. There are no preventive measures, aside from hand hygiene, available for contacts of persons with pneumococcal or viral meningitis.

Exposure to secretions from a potentially rabid animal has been an increasing reason for ED presentation. In part, this has been due to concerns about vaccine and rabies immune globulin (RIG) shortages, and in part visits are often driven by the fear associated with a potential rabies exposure. Excellent overviews of the infection control aspects of rabies are published by the CDC.[47] Although a complete discussion of the indications for rabies prophylaxis vary somewhat geographically and are outside the scope of this chapter, a few general tenets apply. First, if an animal is available for observation or necropsy, no immediate interventions are needed. Second, exposure to bats, foxes, raccoons, skunks, woodchucks, and other wild carnivores should be regarded as rabid and prompt immediate intervention. A comprehensive review of rabies and PEP[48] was published in 2004 and provides an algorithm to assist with the decision to implement prophylaxis.

Quantifying true exposure is one of the greatest challenges in evaluating a child for rabies prophylaxis. This is particularly true given recent shortages of both rabies vaccine and RIG. Assistance for this can often come from local health departments, who can give clinicians data on recent cases of rabies in nonhuman animals, as well as the species most commonly involved. Children with true exposures who are asymptomatic should receive both the rabies vaccine (four total doses) and RIG. RIG should be infiltrated around the wound and, if possible, given concomitantly with the first vaccine dose. If either vaccine or RIG is unavailable, the available product should be given immediately. Persons who previously received the rabies vaccine series should be boosted with two doses of the vaccine, but do not need to receive RIG.[5] If rabies vaccine or RIG is unavailable, contact should be made with the local or state health departments, as in times of shortage, letters from health departments may be necessary to obtain vaccine from manufacturers.

Occasionally, a child presents after exposure to blood—a common scenario might be a toddler who picks up a syringe and needle possibly contaminated by blood. In these circumstances, it is important to obtain baseline serologies for HIV, hepatitis B, and hepatitis C. It is not recommended to test the object to which the child was exposed. These are generally considered very low-risk exposures, to date no cases of HIV transmission have been documented from needles found in the community,[5] and antiretroviral prophylaxis is not indicated. HIV prophylaxis is also not recommended for individuals presenting more than 72 hours after the exposure. If antiretroviral prophylaxis is necessary because of exposure to blood from patients known to have HIV, there are two preferred regimens. The first is protease inhibitor-based [lopinavir/ritonavir + (lamivudine or emtricitabine) + zidovudine] or nonnucleoside reverse transcriptase inhibitor-based [efavirenz + (lamivudine or emtricitabine) + (zidovudine or tenofovir)].[49] The regimen should be continued for four weeks, with appropriate follow-up with an infectious disease physician who can arrange subsequent serologic studies. A four-week course of antiretroviral therapy can often cost more than $1,000, making it prohibitively expensive for many families, and if hospital or other resources are available to defray these costs, these should be sought. The underimmunized child exposed to blood of an individual with hepatitis B should receive both the hepatitis B vaccine and hepatitis B immune globulin (HBIG). HBIG should ideally be given within 24 hours of exposure but remains efficacious until seven days after the exposure. There are no available interventions for the child exposed to hepatitis C.

Health Care Workers

Post-exposure prophylaxis for health care workers tends to occur in two main circumstances: needlestick injuries or other exposures to blood-borne pathogens, and contact with respiratory secretions of patients later found to have meningococcal meningitis. Both are high-stress situations for health care workers and require a systematic approach, readily available infrastructure to provide needed medications, and, if necessary, laboratory testing and reliable communication between employee health services, infection control, and health care workers. The latter is particularly important in the ED, where a patient's ultimate diagnosis is not always known at the time of their disposition from the ED. Many of the recommendations for health care workers parallel those suggested for patients and families with similar exposure histories.

Needlestick injuries and other exposures to blood-borne pathogens are very common in hospital settings. Knowledge of protocols after blood-borne exposures is important in the ED, as this is often where health care workers present after such events when occupational or employee health is closed. Although the risks of contracting HIV and hepatitis C are higher after exposure to blood of adult patients, the evaluation procedure is similar in pediatric EDs. First, the health care worker needs baseline serologies for HIV, hepatitis B, and hepatitis C. As all health care workers should be immunized against hepatitis B, exposure to this pathogen should not be concerning; nonetheless, serologies confirming immunity should be obtained, and if the health care worker is a known nonresponder or has inadequate antibody response, HBIG and hepatitis B vaccine should be administered as soon as possible and preferably within seven days of the exposure. If a health care worker has documented evidence of hepatitis B immunity, no interventions are necessary.[50] No interventions are possible for health care workers exposed to hepatitis C. The health care worker with exposure to bodily fluids of an HIV-infected patient should be started on two- or three-drug antiretroviral therapy for four weeks. One regimen is protease inhibitor-based [lopinavir/ritonavir + (lamivudine or emtricitabine) + zidovudine], while the other recommended regimen is nonnucleoside reverse transcriptase inhibitor-based [efavirenz + (lamivudine or emtricitabine) + (zidovudine or tenofovir)].[49] All health care workers with occupational exposures to blood-borne pathogens should be referred to occupational health for additional testing.

It is common for health care workers in pediatric EDs to be exposed to children with pertussis. If the diagnosis is suspected in the ED, the patient should be placed in a private room with droplet precautions (mask, gown) used by health care workers. Often, however, the diagnosis is only suspected after a health care worker is exposed to a child with pertussis. In these instances, azithromycin (five-day course), clarithromycin (seven-day course), or trimethoprim-sulfamethoxazole (14-day course) provide effective chemoprophylaxis. Although health care workers (and other adults) are encouraged to receive the TDaP vaccine for booster doses, receipt of this vaccine does not eliminate the need to receive chemoprophylaxis.[17]

Another common scenario is the health care worker exposed to the child with possible meningococcal meningitis. Droplet precautions should be used for children with suspected meningococcal disease, but if a health care worker has significant contact with patient secretions

TABLE 5-6

Common Infections for Which Health Care Workers Should Be Excluded from Patient Care Responsibilities

Infection	Time Excluded From Patient Care
Abscess/cellulitis	Until on appropriate antibiotics and wound no longer draining, if it cannot be covered
Adenoviral conjunctivitis	14 days after disease onset in the most recently involved eye
Diarrhea	If incontinent, until resolution of symptoms; otherwise, can continue to work with contact precautions
Hepatitis A	1 week after symptom onset
Herpes Simplex Virus	Cold sores: cover and do not touch mouth Whitlow: cover; no contact with neonates or immuno-compromised hosts until lesion is healed
Measles	4 days after rash develops
Mumps	9 days after symptom onset
Pertussis	If treated: 5 days after begin therapy If untreated: 21 days from onset of cough
Rubella	5 days after rash appears
SARS	If exposed, isolate for 10 days.
Streptococcus, Group A	24 hours after start of antibiotic therapy
Tuberculosis	Until effective therapy initiated, AFB sputum smears have become negative, and cough has abated
Varicella	5 days after rash onset and until all lesions are crusted
Zoster	Contact precautions until all lesions are crusted; exclude from work if lesions cannot be covered

AFB – acid fast baccillus

Adapted from American Academy of Pediatrics. Pickering L.K., (ed.): *2006 Red Book: Report of the Committee on Infectious Diseases.* 27th ed. Elk Grove Village, IL: American Academy of Pediatrics; 2006.

(e.g., intubation, suctioning) without a mask, chemoprophylaxis should be offered. Rifampin (600 mg twice daily for two days), ceftriaxone (250 mg single intramuscular dose), or ciprofloxacin (500 mg single dose) are equally efficacious and should be given immediately after the diagnosis is confirmed or suspected; the efficacy of chemoprophylaxis begun 14 or more days after exposure is unknown.[5] Chemoprophylaxis is neither recommended nor available for pneumococcal or viral meningitis.

Indications for Excluding a Health Care Worker from Work

There are circumstances under which health care workers should be excluded from patient care responsibilities until they have resolution of symptoms. Some are due to specific etiologic diagnoses (Table 5-6, above), while others are due to symptomatology (conjunctivitis, diarrhea). For many mild illnesses (such as upper respiratory tract infections), use of hand hygiene and barrier (contact)

TABLE 5-7

Recommendations for Return to Work for Health Care Workers Susceptible to Measles, Mumps, Rubella, and Varicella in Times of Community Outbreaks and Direct Contact with Affected Patient

Disease	Ill?	Acute Interventions	Return to Work Criteria
Measles	Yes	None	4 days after rash develops
	No	Immunoglobulin (IG) within 6 days of exposure and/or vaccine within 3 days of exposure	5th day after first exposure to 21st day after last exposure, regardless if had receipt of vaccine or immunoglobulin
Mumps	Yes	None	9 days after symptom onset
	No	Vaccine can be given, but questionable efficacy	12th day after first exposure to 26th day after last exposure
Rubella	Yes	None	5 days after rash appears
	No	Vaccine within 3 days of exposure (theoretical benefit)	7th day after first exposure to 21st day after last exposure
Varicella	Yes	Consider acyclovir; IG and vaccine not indicated after symptom onset	Minimum of 5 days after rash onset and until all lesions are crusted
	No	Varicella vaccine within 3–5 days after exposure; IG up to 4 days after exposure. Consider acyclovir in immunocompromised hosts if IG unavailable	Received IG: 10th to 28th day after exposure Did not receive IG: 10th to 21st day after exposure

Adapted from American Academy of Pediatrics. Pickering L.K., (ed.): *2006 Red Book: Report of the Committee on Infectious Diseases.* 27th ed. Elk Grove Village, IL: American Academy of Pediatrics, 2006.

Centers for Disease Control and Prevention. Measles, mumps, and rubella—vaccine use and strategies for elimination of measles, rubella, and congenital rubella syndrome and control of mumps: recommendations of the Advisory Committee on Immunization Practices (ACIP). *MMWR* 47(No. RR-8), 1998.

precautions can enable health care workers to continue to work while minimizing risk to their patients. During a pandemic, the exclusion of affected health care workers can limit the ability of health care organizations to serve patient needs in key locations, such as the ED. This observation during the 2009 H1N1 event led to a reduction in the CDC's recommended exclusion period for ill health care providers.

The Under-Immunized Health Care Worker During Epidemics or After Contact With an Infected Child

There is no mandatory vaccination of health care workers, and it is estimated that well over one-third of employees engaged in patient care at hospitals are not immunized to at least one of the recommended vaccines.[51] This leads to a significant cohort of potentially susceptible health care workers, which is of particular concern for measles and varicella, which are highly transmissible and immunization levels over 90% are needed to confer herd immunity. Although compulsory vaccination cannot be implemented, health care workers who are not immunized or immune to certain infections can be held out of work during outbreaks of particular diseases or after contact with patients with these illnesses. The recommendations of the CDC and the AAP are summarized in Table 5-7, page 91.

References

1. Centers for Disease Control and Prevention: Guideline for hand hygiene in health-care settings. *MMWR* 51:1–56, 2002.
2. Klevens R.M., Edwards J.R., Richards C.L., et al.: Estimating health care-associated infections and deaths in U.S. hospitals, 2002. *Public Health Rep* 122:160–166, 2007.
3. Pessoa-Silva C.L., Hugonnet S., Pfister R., et al.: Reduction of healthcare-associated infection risk in neonates by successful hand hygiene promotion. *Pediatrics* 120:e382–390, 2007.
4. Siegel J.D., Rhinehart E., Jackson M., Chairello L., and the Healthcare Infection Control Practices Advisory Committee: 2007 Guideline for isolation precautions: preventing transmission of infectious agents in healthcare settings. June 2007. http://www.cdc.gov/ncidod/dhqp/pdf/isolation2007.pdf.
5. American Academy of Pediatrics. Pickering L.K. (ed.): *2006 Red Book: Report of the Committee on Infectious Diseases.* 27th ed. Elk Grove Village, IL: American Academy of Pediatrics, 2006.
6. Centers for Disease Control and Prevention: Infection control in healthcare settings. http://www.cdc.gov/ncidod/dhqp/index.html (accessed Aug. 27, 2008).
7. Johnston C.P., Qiu H., Ticehurst J.R., et al.: Outbreak management and implications of a nosocomial norovirus outbreak. *Clin Infect Dis* 45:534–540, 2007.
8. Centers for Disease Control and Prevention: Brief report: respiratory syncytial virus activity—United States, 2005–2006. *MMWR* 55:1277–1279, 2006.
9. Hall C.B.: Nosocomial respiratory syncytial virus infections: the 'Cold War' has not ended. *Clin Infect Dis* 31:590–596, 2000.
10. Groothuis J., Bauman J., Malinoski F., Eggleston M.: Strategies for prevention of RSV nosocomial infection. *J Perinatol* 28:319–323, 2008.
11. American Academy of Pediatrics, Committee on Infectious Disease, Subcommittee on Diagnosis and Management of Bronchiolitis: Diagnosis and management of bronchiolitis. *Pediatrics* 118:1774–1793, 2006.
12. Pont S.J., Carpenter L.R., Griffin M.R., et al.: Trends in healthcare usage attributable to diarrhea, 1995–2004. *J Pediatr,* Aug 8 [Epub ahead of print], 2008.
13. Vernacchio L., Vezina R.M., Mitchell A.A., et al.: Diarrhea in American infants and young children in the community setting: incidence, clinical presentation and microbiology. *Pediatr Infect Dis* J 25:2–7, 2006.
14. Van Damme P., Giaquinto C., Huet F., et al., REVEAL Study Group: Multicenter prospective study of the burden of rotavirus acute gastroenteritis in Europe, 2004–2005: the REVEAL study. *J Infect Dis* 195 (Suppl 1): S4–S16, 2007.
15. Kaplan S.L., Hulten K.G., Gonzalez B.E., et al.: Three-year surveillance of community-acquired *Staphylococcus aureus* infections in children. *Clin Infect Dis* 40:1785–1791, 2005.
16. Centers for Disease Control and Prevention: Personal protective equipment (PPE) in healthcare settings. http://www.cdc.gov/ncidod/dhqp/ppe.html (accessed Aug. 30, 2008).
17. Centers for Disease Control and Prevention. Vaccinations for healthcare workers http://www.cdc.gov/vaccines/spec-grps/hcw.htm (accessed Aug. 30, 2008).
18. Meyer C.U., Zepp F., Decker M., et al.: Cellular immunity in adolescents and adults following acellular pertussis administration. *Clin Vaccine Immunol* 14:288–292, 2007.
19. Glezen W.P.: Modifying clinical practices to manage influenza in children effectively. *Pediatr Infect Dis* 27:738–743, 2008.
20. Talan D.A., Moran G.J., Mower W.R., et al.: EMERGEncy ID NET: an emergency department-based emerging infections sentinel network. *Ann Emerg Med* 32:703–711, 1998.
21. Wu T.S., Shih F.Y., Yen M.Y., et al.: Establishing a nationwide emergency department-based syndromic surveillance system for better public health responses in Taiwan. *BMC Public Health* 8:18–31, 2008.
22. Brillman J.C., Burr T., Forslund D., et al.: Modeling emergency department visit patterns for infectious disease complaints: results and application to disease surveillance. *BMC Med Informatics Decision Making* 5:4–18, 2005.
23. Centers for Disease Control and Prevention: Nationally notifiable diseases, 2008. www.cdc.gov/epo/dphsi/phs/infdis.htm (accessed Aug. 30, 2008).
24. Srinivasan A., McDonald L.C., Jernigan D., et al.: SARS Healthcare Preparedness and Response Plan Team. Foundations of the severe acute respiratory syndrome preparedness and response plan for healthcare facilities. *Infect Control Hosp Epidemiol* 25:1020–1025, 2004.
25. Ollerton J.E.: Emergency department response to the deliberate release of biological agents. *Emerg Med J* 21:5–8, 2004.
26. Centers for Disease Control and Prevention: http://www.bt.cdc.gov/agent/agentlist (accessed Sep. 1, 2008).
27. Tham K.Y.: An emergency department response to severe acute respiratory syndrome: a prototype response to bioterrorism. *Ann Emerg Med* 43:6–14, 2004.
28. Filoromo C., Macrina D., Pryor E., et al.: An innovative approach to training hospital-based clinicians for bioterrorist attacks. *Am J Infect Control* 31:511–114, Dec. 2003.
29. Patt H.A., Feigin R.D.: Diagnosis and management of suspected cases of bioterrorism: a pediatric perspective. *Pediatrics* 109: 685–692, 2002.
30. Kman N.E., Nelson R.N.: Infectious agents of bioterrorism: a review for emergency physicians. *Emerg Med Clin North Am* 26:517–547, 2008.
31. Centers for Disease Control and Prevention: Prevention and control of influenza: recommendations of the Advisory Committee on Immunization Practices (ACIP), 2008. *MMWR* 57:1–60, 2008.
32. Patriarca P.A., Cox N.J.: Influenza pandemic preparedness plan for the United States. *J Infect Dis* 176:S4–S7, 1997.
33. Turnberg W., Daniell W., Seixas N., et al.: Appraisal of recommended respiratory infection control practices in primary care and emergency department settings. *Am J Infect Control* 36:268–275, 2008.

34. Swaminathan A., Martin R., Gamon S., et al.: Personal protective equipment and antiviral drug use during hospitalization for suspected avian or pandemic influenza. *Emerg Infect Dis* 13:1541–1547, 2007.

35. Harrison P.F., Lederberg J. (eds.): *Antimicrobial Resistance: Issues and Options. Workshop Report.* In: Washington, D.C.: National Academy Press; 1998.

36. Ongkasuwan J., Valdez T.A., Hulten K.G., et al.: Pneumococcal mastoiditis in children and the emergence of multidrug-resistant serotype 19A isolates. *Pediatrics* 122:34–9, Jul. 2008.

37. Denton M., Kerr K., Mooney L., et al.: Transmission of colistin-resistant Pseudomonas aeruginosa between patients attending a pediatric cystic fibrosis center. *Pediatr Pulmonol* 34:257–261, 2002.

38. Siegel J.D., Rhinehart E., Jackson M., Chairello L., and the Healthcare Infection Control Practices Advisory Committee: Management of multidrug-resistant organisms in healthcare settings, 2006. http://www.cdc.gov/ncidod/dhqp/pdf/ar/mdroGuideline2006.pdf.

39. Aboelela S.W., Saiman L., Stone P., et al.: Effectiveness of barrier precautions and surveillance cultures to control transmission of multidrug-resistant organisms: a systematic review of the literature. *Am J Infect Control* 34:484–494, 2006.

40. Lidsky K., Hoyen C., Salvator A., et al.: Antibiotic-resistant Gram-negative organisms in pediatric chronic-care facilities. *Clin Infect Dis* 34:760–6, 2002.

41. Cordery R.J., Roberts C.H., Cooper S.J., et al.: Evaluation of risk factors for the acquisition of bloodstream infections with extended-spectrum-lactamase-producing *E. coli* and *Klebsiella* species in the intensive care unit; antibiotic management and clinical outcome. *J Hosp Infect* 68:108–115, 2008.

42. Jensen P.A., Lambert L.A., Iademarco M.F., Ridzen R.: Guidelines for preventing the transmission of tuberculosis in healthcare settings: 2005. *MMWR* 54:1–141, 2005.

43. Centers for Disease Control and Prevention. www.cdc.gov/od/ohs/biosfty/bmbl5/sections/AppendixB.pdf.

44. Hall L., Otter J.A., Chewins J., Wegenack N.L.: Use of hydrogen peroxide vapor for deactivation of Mycobacterium tuberculosis in a biological safety cabinet and a room. *J Clin Microbiol* 45:810–815, 2007.

45. Muñoz F.M., Ong L.T., Seavy D., et al.: Tuberculosis among adult visitors of children with suspected tuberculosis and employees at a children's hospital. *Infect Control Hosp Epidemiol* 23:568–572, 2002.

46. Moran G.J., Fuchs M.A., Jarvis W.R., Talan D.A.: Tuberculosis infection-control practices in United States emergency departments. *Ann Emerg Med* 26:283–289, 1995.

47. Manning S.E., Rupprecht C.E., Fishbein D., et al.; Advisory Committee on Immunization Practices, Centers for Disease Control and Prevention (CDC): Human rabies prevention—United States, 2008: recommendations of the Advisory Committee on Immunization Practices. *MMWR Recomm Rep* 57(RR-3):1–28, May 23, 2008.

48. Rupprecht C.E., Gibbons R.V.: Clinical practice. Prophylaxis against rabies. *N Engl J Med* 351:2626–2635, 2004.

49. Centers for Disease Control and Prevention: Antiretroviral post-exposure prophylaxis after sexual, injection drug use, or other nonoccupational exposure to HIV in the United States. *MMWR* 54:1–20, 2005.

50. Centers for Disease Control and Prevention: Updated U.S. Public Health Service Guidelines for the Management of Occupational Exposures to HBV, HCV, and HIV and Recommendations for Postexposure Prophylaxis. *MMWR* 50:1–42, 2001.

51. Calderon M., Feja K.N., Ford P., et al.: Implementation of a pertussis immunization program in a teaching hospital: an argument for federally mandated pertussis vaccination of health care workers. *Am J Infect Control* 36:392–398, 2008.

52. Centers for Disease Control and Prevention: Measles, mumps, and rubella—vaccine use and strategies for elimination of measles, rubella, and congenital rubella syndrome and control of mumps: recommendations of the Advisory Committee on Immunization Practices (ACIP). *MMWR* 47(No. RR-8), 1998.

CHAPTER 6

Pediatric Patient Assessment, Diagnostic Studies, and Treatment in the ED

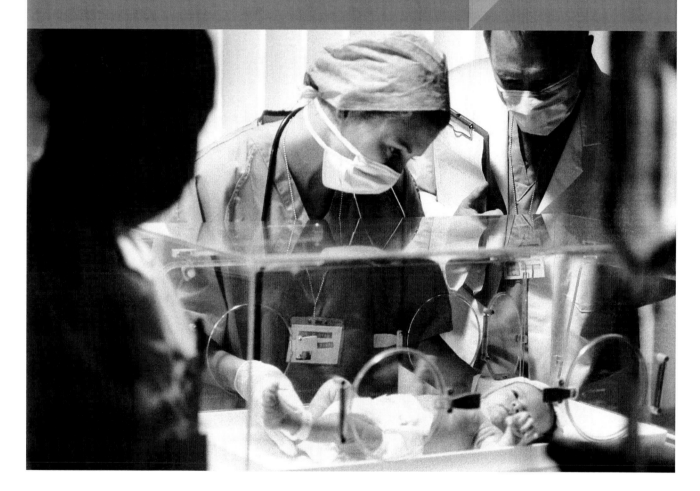

Authored by Steven E. Krug, M.D., F.A.A.P., *Head of the Division of Emergency Medicine, Children's Memorial Hospital, Chicago*

There are many challenges associated with providing optimal care for children in the emergency department (ED) setting. These challenges are the direct result of the unique anatomic, physiologic, behavioral, and developmental characteristics of children and their related care needs. As some emergency care providers may not possess sufficient training or experience concerning the unique illnesses and injuries that are specific to the pediatric population, or, more importantly, may practice in a setting where they do not have adequate ongoing clinical exposure to children, they could be at risk for errors in their approach to assessment or treatment of pediatric patients.[1] Although children represent approximately one quarter of all patient visits to EDs, 50% of EDs in the United States care for 10 or less children daily.[2]

As medical research and advances in technology have contributed to the knowledge base and practice of emergency medicine, the vast majority of these advances, and most of the related research, have focused on adult populations.[1] In the absence of sufficient medical evidence in pediatric populations, there has been a logical tendency to extrapolate well accepted, and at times, evidence-based, adult patient care practices to children. Some of these same diagnostic testing practices have also been fueled by concerns related to professional risk with an intention to reduce medical liability.

Clinicians bear an important responsibility to employ diagnostic testing and treatment modalities with discretion as the sensitivity and specificity of laboratory studies and medical imaging in children, and the risks associated with these tests, may be different than that in adult patients. The same risk/benefit considerations also apply to therapeutic interventions. This chapter emphasizes the importance of understanding the differences between children and adults and offers a perspective on the customization of the emergency care process for pediatric patients. The chapter also reviews some important examples where the relative benefit and risk of diagnostic testing in children deserve thoughtful consideration. The chapter also emphasizes the importance of ED preparedness for pediatric patients, using trauma as an example, and considerations for the interfacility transfer of critically ill and injured children. Finally, the chapter acknowledges the essential safety-net role of the ED, and the need for vigilance and the ability to screen for maltreatment and mental health emergencies in children and adolescents.

Customizing the Emergency Care Process for Children

The statement "children are not little adults" is often used to convey the fact that children have unique health care needs relative to adults. In fact, the anatomical, physiological, developmental, and emotional attributes of children impact not only their susceptibility to illness and injury but also the ways in which providers need to assess and treat them.[1] In "customizing" the care provided to children in the ED, consideration should be given to all steps within the emergency care process, including triage,

patient evaluation, diagnostic testing, and disposition (discharge home, observation, admission, transfer to a tertiary center).

Triage is an essential first encounter with patients presenting for emergency care as it informs the ED care team of the relative acuity of patients who have not yet been fully evaluated and supports the appropriate prioritization of fixed resources (e.g., space, staff, ancillary services). Accurate and efficient triage systems have become increasingly important with the growing prevalence of ED overcrowding. Unfortunately, some general patient acuity scoring systems or triage tools may not apply well to children of all ages or to children with special care needs. Combined with limited ongoing exposure to the unique signs of serious illness in children for many ED staff,[2,3] this could result in an inaccurate triage assessment of the pediatric patient. Whether the outcome is the under-assessment of a severely ill child, or the "over-triage" of children with minor illnesses, both represent suboptimal performance that could pose a patient safety concern for the index patient, or for others in the ED from whom limited resources are diverted.

Therefore, an important first step in preparing for pediatric patients is to assure that the ED triage scoring system incorporates pediatric-specific criteria (e.g., age-based vital signs, chief complaints), and that the clinical staff have ongoing professional education in pediatric assessment and opportunities to practice this important clinical function. As recommended by the American Academy of Pediatrics (AAP), the American College of Emergency Physicians (ACEP), and the Emergency Nurses Association (ENA) in their joint policy statement addressing guidelines for the care of pediatric patients in the ED, baseline and periodic competency evaluations should be completed for all ED clinical staff, including physicians.[3] These competency evaluations should be age-specific and include neonates, infants, children, and adolescents, and children with special health care needs. Sidebar 6-1, page 97, contains an appendix from that policy statement offering some suggested topics for clinical and professional competency assessment.

In assessing the pediatric patient, one must remember that there are unique characteristics for several somewhat distinct age-related subgroups, including: neonates (0–28 days); infants (1–12 months); toddlers (1–3 years); pre-school-aged (3–6 years); school-aged (6–12 years); and adolescents (12–18 years). What is considered to be a normal heart rate, respiratory rate, or blood pressure varies

Sidebar 6-1 | **Clinical and Professional Competency**

Demonstration and maintenance of pediatric clinical competency may be achieved through a number of continuing education mechanisms, including participation in local educational programs, professional organization conferences, and national life-support programs (such as Pediatric Advanced Life Support,[1] Advanced Pediatric Life Support: The Pediatric Emergency Medicine Course,[2] Emergency Nurses Pediatric Course[3]) or through scheduled mock codes or patient simulation, team training exercises, or experiences in other clinical settings, such as the operating room (i.e., airway management).

Potential areas for the development of pediatric competency and professional performance evaluations may include but should not be limited to:

1. Triage
2. Illness and injury assessment and management
3. Pain assessment and treatment, including sedation and analgesia
4. Airway management
5. Vascular access
6. Critical care monitoring
7. Neonatal and pediatric resuscitation
8. Trauma care
9. Burn care
10. Mass-casualty events
11. Patient- and family-centered care
12. Medication delivery and device/equipment safety
13. Team training and effective communication

References

1. Ralston M., Hazinski M.F., Zaritsky A.L., et al. (eds.); American Heart Association and American Academy of Pediatrics : PALS Course Guide and PALS Provider Manual: Provider Manual. Dallas, TX: American Heart Association, 2007. ISBN-10: 0874935288, ISBN-13: 9780874935288.
2. Gausche-Hill M., Fuchs S., Yamamoto L. (eds.): APLS: The Pediatric Emergency Medicine Resource—4th Ed. Sudbury, MA: Jones and Bartlett, 2004.
3. Emergency Nurses Association. Emergency Nursing Pediatric Course. Available at: http://www.ena.org/catn_enpc_tncc/enpc/ (accessed Feb. 5, 2009).

American Academy of Pediatrics Committee on Pediatric Emergency Medicine, American College of Emergency Physicians Pediatric Committee, Emergency Nurses Association Pediatric Committee: Guidelines for care of children in the emergency department. *Pediatrics* 124: 1233-1243, Oct. 2009. Printed with permission.

widely with a child's age and weight. Heart rate and respiratory rate typically decline with age, while systolic blood pressure increases with age. Table 6-1, page 98, is an example of a pediatric vital sign reference that can be found in many pediatric emergency care textbooks, and such a resource may prove to be useful in assisting ED staff in their determination of whether or not a child's vital signs are normal.

Evaluation of the pediatric patient obviously goes beyond the vital signs and should be built upon a reliable initial assessment. For many pediatric patients, especially the most developmentally immature, this may also require some special assessment techniques. Both the Advanced Pediatric Life Support (APLS)[4] and the Pediatric Education for Prehospital Professionals (PEPP)[5] courses recommend the Pediatric Assessment Triangle (PAT) as a simple and consistent approach to the development of a general impression regarding the acutely ill or injured child.

The PAT (see Figure 6-1, page 98) is based on three components: appearance, work of breathing, and circulation to the skin. Combining the information from these three components of the PAT may allow the clinician to determine the most likely physiologic abnormality, the severity of the child's illness or injury, and how quickly one must intervene.

For ED care providers who may be more experienced and comfortable in the assessment and care of adult patients, construction of an accurate pediatric assessment and the determination of a care plan require consideration of the anatomical, physiological, developmental, and emotional differences between children and adults. Examples of these differences are listed in Table 6-2, page 99.[1]

The age and developmental stage of the pediatric patient may also impose unique behavioral characteristics that require special assessment techniques for the gathering of

TABLE 6-1

Vital Signs: What's Normal for Kids

What is considered a normal heart rate, blood pressure, and respiratory rate varies widely with a child's age and weight. Heart rate and respiratory rate typically decline with age, while systolic BP increases with age. Here are some general ranges to keep in mind:

Age	Heart rate (beats/min)	Systolic BP* (mm Hg)	Respiration (breaths/min)
Neonate	100–180	40–80	30–50
Infant	100–160	60–80	30–40
Toddler	90–150	70–90	24–36
Pre-school age	80–140	75–100	22–30
School-age	70–120	80–110	18–24
Adolescent	60–110	90–120	12–20

* Normal diastolic blood pressure is two-thirds that of systolic pressure.

Adapted from Gunn V.L., Nechyba C.: *The Harriet Lane Handbook: A Manual for Pediatric House Officers,* Sixteenth Edition. Philadelphia, PA: Mosby, 2002, pp. 136, 513.

Pediatric Assessment: Normal vital signs for children of various age groups. Emergency Medical Services for Children. New Jersey Department of Health and Senior Services, June 2005.

FIGURE 6-1

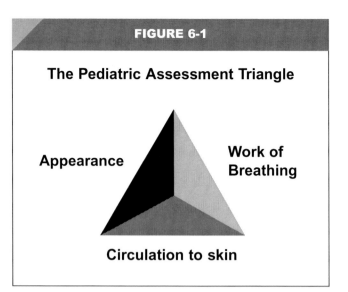

The Pediatric Assessment Triangle

Gausche-Hill M., Fuchs S., Yamamoto L. (eds.): *APLS: The Pediatric Emergency Medicine Resource,* Revised Fourth Edition, Sudbury, MD: Jones and Bartlett, 2007. Printed with permission.

In addition to their unique physical and psychological attributes, children are also not little adults from an epidemiology and prevalence of disease perspective. Children possess a scope of illnesses and injuries that are unique to them. In fact, these disorders may be specific to age-based sub-populations of children. There are many examples of this essential difference between pediatric and adult patients. A presenting complaint of chest pain in an adult will typically prompt an emergent assessment for a cardiovascular etiology. In the pediatric population, chest pain is a fairly uncommon presenting symptom and, in the absence of certain risk factors (e.g., congenital heart disease, sickle cell anemia), is rarely due to cardiac disease and is more likely secondary to respiratory illness or may be musculoskeletal in origin.

Abdominal pain is a much more common presenting complaint for children and provides an excellent example of both the broad range of potential causes and age group-specific differential diagnoses in the pediatric population. As is demonstrated in Table 6-4, page 102,[6] although gastroenteritis may be a common cause of pain in all age groups, there are specific entities that are characteristic for infant, pre-school, school-age, and adolescent age groups. Appendicitis can be found in all age groups but is quite uncommon in infants and pre-school aged children. Likewise, certain structural causes, such as intussusception and volvulus, present more commonly in infants and toddlers.

Assessing the presence of key symptoms such as abdominal pain can be extremely challenging in younger age groups. Likewise, infants and young children may poorly localize

clinical data (see Table 6-3, page 101). These techniques may be particularly helpful when caring for younger children, who may not routinely cooperate with a clinical exam. As an example, for patients (e.g., toddlers and pre-school aged children) where there may be a very narrow window of opportunity in terms of "quiet cooperation" with the exam, the most essential exam components, and particularly those that are best done while the child is not crying, should be pursued first. Likewise, components that may be invasive or unwelcome, such as the examination of the oropharynx or ears, should be left for last. Whenever possible, children are best examined in a location or "position of comfort," which for many may represent their parents' lap.

TABLE 6-2

Examples of Differences Between Children and Adults and Implications for Care

	Pediatric Characteristic	Implications for Illness and Injury	Implications for Care
Anatomical Differences	Greater surface area relative to body volume.	Greater risk of excessive loss of heat and fluids; children are affected more quickly and easily by toxins that are absorbed through the skin.	Increased body surface area makes children more susceptible to greater heat loss when they are exposed during resuscitation; the higher percentage of body surface area devoted to the head relative to the lower extremities must be taken into account when determining the percentage of body surface area involved in burn injuries.
	Smaller airways; tongue is large relative to the oropharynx; larynx is higher and more anterior in the neck; vocal cords are at a more anterocaudal angle; epiglottis is soft and shaped differently from that in adults.	A right main stem intubation can lead to iatrogenic complications; more susceptible to respiratory distress due to airway swelling from infection or inflammation.	Special equipment and training are needed for intubation; appropriately sized endotracheal intubation tubes, stylettes, and laryngoscope blades are necessary. A child's airway is more difficult to maintain and intubate. Children are at higher risk for a right mainstem bronchus intubation.
	Less protective muscle around internal organs.	Internal organs are more susceptible to traumatic forces.	Recognition of internal injury requires a high degree of suspicion, and such injury should not be ruled out based on the absence of external signs of trauma.
	Small size.	More vulnerable to exposure and toxicity from agents that are heavier than air, such as sarin gas and chlorine, and that accumulate closer to the ground.	
	Less fat, less elastic connective tissue, and closer proximity of chest and abdominal organs.	Higher frequency of multiple organ injury.	
	Head is proportionally larger and heavier in children.	Head injury is common in young children.	Head size also makes children more susceptible to greater heat loss when they are exposed during resuscitation.
	More pliable skeleton with growth plates; thoracic cage of a child does not provide as much protection of organs as that of adults.	More susceptible to fracture and other injuries from blunt trauma.	Orthopedic injuries with subtle symptoms are easily missed; hepatic or splenic injuries can go unrecognized and produce significant blood loss, leading to shock.

(Continued on next page)

TABLE 6-2

Examples of Differences Between Children
and Adults and Implications for Care *(continued)*

	Pediatric Characteristic	Implications for Illness and Injury	Implications for Care
Physiological Differences	More rapid respiratory and heart rates that vary with age.	More susceptible to airborne toxins.	Knowledge of normal and abnormal rates based on age is required; normal vital signs differ for children and adults. An increased heart rate is often the first sign of shock in a pediatric patient, versus blood pressure in an adult. Children maintain heart rate during the early phases of hypovolemic shock, creating a false impression of normalcy.
	Higher metabolic rates.	More susceptible to contaminants in food or water; greater risk for increased loss of fluid when ill or stressed.	Medication doses must be carefully calculated based on the child's weight and body size.
	Lower blood pressure levels than adults; levels vary with age.		Indicators of serious illness may not appear until the child is near collapse. Vital signs are less reliable indicators of serious illness than in adults. Respiratory arrest is more common than cardiac arrest; cardio-pulmonary arrest is signaled by respiratory arrest or shock, rather than by cardiac arrhythmias.
	Immature immunological systems.	Greater risk of infection; less herd immunity from infections such as smallpox.	
Developmental Differences	Communication barriers may exist in all pediatric age groups, but the nature of the barrier varies by age (infants and young children cannot articulate symptoms).		Assessment tools need to be tailored to reflect age-appropriate responses.
Emotional Differences	Greater, varying emotional needs based on developmental level.		Need for family-centered policies and a family-friendly environment in EDs. Depending on age, children require or prefer the presence of a parent during treatment.
	Higher sensitivity to environmental factors during treatment.	Age and developmental level of child, characteristics of event, and parental reactions play significant roles in determining the child's reactions and recovery.	Providers must manage the mental health needs of pediatric patients and parents' reactions.

Adapted from Institute of Medicine, Committee on the Future of Emergency Care in the U.S. Health System. Emergency Care for Children: Growing Pains. Washington, D.C.: National Academies Press, 2006. Table 1-1, pp. 18–21. Table reprinted with permission.

TABLE 6-3

Behavioral Characteristics and Special Assessment Techniques

Developmental Age	Behavioral Characteristics	Special Assessment Techniques
Neonate	Primitive reflexes only	Immediately assess airway, breathing, heart rate, and color. Because the neonate has no interactive behavior yet, focus assessment of appearance on muscle tone, spontaneous motor activity, and quality of cry.
Infant Under 2 months	Physiologic responses No separation anxiety	Obtain the pregnancy and delivery history, because manifestation of intrapartum or perinatal disease often manifest in this age. Signs of serious illness might be nonspecific, so a history of fussiness, feeding difficulty, or poor sleeping can be significant symptom of sepsis, metabolic abnormality, or a central nervous system problem. An episode of choking, apnea, loss of tone, or change in skin color might represent an apparent life-threatening event, or ALTE. Examine in any position.
2–6 months	Social skills (smiles, tracks), motor skills (rolls over, sits, reaches), and vocalization	As infants develop a wider range of behaviors and become more interactive with the environment, TICLS as a measure of appearance becomes a more reliable indicator of disease and injury. Examine in any position and use distraction. Use calm, lilting speech to soothe and engage child.
6–12 months	Socially interactive Stranger/separation anxiety Sits without support Plays, babbles	Leave child on caregiver's lap. Anticipate stranger anxiety. Sit or squat at child's level. Offer toys and distractions (tongue blade, penlight). Examine toe-to-head.
Toddler	Fearless curiosity Strong opinions, illogical Egocentrism Stranger/separation anxiety Wide verbal variability	Approach gently and observe from the doorway. Leave the child on the caregiver's lap and get down to the child's level. Enlist the caregiver's assistance. Use distraction. Talk to the child about herself. Employ endless praise and reassurance. Explain procedures simply. Do the exam toe-to-head.
Preschooler	Magical, illogical thinkers Misconceptions about illness and injury but logical Fears of mutilation, loss of control, death, darkness, and being alone Good language skills Examine health-to-toe	Speak directly to the child. Choose words carefully and clarify misconceptions. Use dolls or puppets for explanation. Allow the child to handle equipment and ask for her help. Set limits on behavior. Use games and distractions. Praise cooperation and avoid ridicule.
School-aged Child	Talkative, analytical Understand cause and effect Want involvement in care Fears of separation, loss of control, pain, and physical disability	Speak directly to child and provide simple explanations. Anticipate questions and fears. Explain procedures and never lie. Respect privacy. Do not negotiate but provide options. Involve the child in the treatment.
Adolescent	Mobile, experimental, illogical Understand cause and effect Expressive Fears of loss of independence, loss of control, body image	Explain everything. Encourage questions. Show respect and speak directly to patient. Be honest and nonjudgemental. Honor modesty and confidentiality. Do not succumb to provocation. Ask friends for assistance.
Child with Special Health Care Needs	Developmental age can be quite different than chronological age. Child might represent mix of physical and emotional abnormalities.	Use understanding language and techniques. Do not assume the child is mentally impaired. Use information from caregiver and physician when possible.

Gausche-Hill M., Fuchs S., Yamamoto L. (eds.): *APLS: The Pediatric Emergency Medicine Resource,* Revised Fourth Edition, Sudbury, MD: Jones and Bartlett, 2007. Printed with permission.

pain complaints. Pain from a variety of intra-abdominal sources in younger children is frequently reported to be peri-umbilical in location, and inflammatory processes involving extra-abdominal structures (e.g., pneumonia, pharyngitis) may also present as abdominal pain. Maintaining an awareness of these key developmental and physiologic characteristics, and age-range specific disease pathogenesis, may also drive diagnostic testing that is specific to a particular disease entity such as an ultrasound or contrast enema in infants and toddlers with abdominal pain suspected of having intussusception. The use of pediatric-specific chief-complaint-driven clinical guidelines may prove to be useful in guiding the evaluation and diagnostic assessment of children presenting to the ED.

TABLE 6-4

Causes of Acute Abdoominal Pain

Infancy (<2 yr)	Preschool Age (2–5 yr)	School Age (>5 yr)	Adolescent
Colic (age <3 mo)	Acute gastroenteritis	Acute gastroenteritis	Acute gastroenteritis
Gastroesophageal reflux disease (GERD)	Urinary tract infection (UTI)	Trauma	Gastritis (primary or alcohol induced)
Acute gastroenteritis	Trauma	Appendicitis	Colitis (food intolerance)
"Viral syndromes"	Appendicitis	UTI	GERD
	Pneumonia, asthma	Functional abdominal pain	Trauma
	Sickling syndromes	Sickling syndromes	Constipation
	"Viral syndromes"	Constipation	Appendicitis
	Constipation	"Viral syndromes"	Pelvic inflammatory disease
			UTI
			Pneumonia, bronchitis, asthma
			"Viral syndromes"
			Dysmenorrhea
			Epididymitis
			Lactose intolerance
			Sickling syndromes
			Mittelschmerz

Less Common

Trauma (possible child abuse)	Meckel's diverticulum	Pneumonia, asthma, cystic fibrosis	Ectopic pregnancy
Intussusception	Henoch-Schönlein purpura (anaphylactoid purpura)	Inflammatory bowel disease	Testicular torsion
Intestinal anomalies	Toxin	Peptic ulcer disease	Ovarian torsion
Incarcerated hernia	Cystic fibrosis	Cholecystitis, pancreatic disease	Renal calculi
Sickling syndromes	Intussusception	Diabetes mellitus	Peptic ulcer disease
Milk protein allergy	Nephrotic syndrome	Collagen vascular disease	Hepatitis
		Testicular torsion	Cholecystitis or pancreatic disease
			Meconium-ileus equivalent (cystic fibrosis)
			Collagen vascular disease
			Inflammatory bowel disease
			Toxin

Very Uncommon or Rare

Appendicitis	Incarcerated hernia	Rheumatic fever, myocarditis, pericarditis	Rheumatic fever
Volvulus	Neoplasm	Hepatitis	Toxin
Tumors (e.g., Wilms')	Hemolytic uremic syndrome	Inflammatory bowel disease	Renal calculi
Toxin (heavy metal—PB)		Choledochal cyst	Tumor
Disaccharidase deficiency		Hemolytic anemia	Ovarian torsion
Malabsorptive syndromes		Diabetes mellitus	Meconium-ileus equivalent (cystic fibrosis)
		Porphyria	Intussusception
			Pyomositis of abdomen
			Rheumatic fever
			Tumor
			Abdominal abscess

Source: Ruddy R.M.: Abdominal pain. In Fleisher G.R., Ludwig S., Henretig F.M., Ruddy R., Silverman B.K. (eds.): *Textbook of Pediatric Emergency Medicine—5th ed.* Philadelphia, PA: Lippincott, Williams & Wilkins, 2006, pp. 469–476. [Table 50.1, p. 470.] Printed with permission.

Determining When to Proceed With Diagnostic Testing

When ED practices based on the epidemiology and mechanism of illness and injury in adult patients are applied to the emergency care of children, these practices not only run the risk of misdiagnosis but also unnecessary testing procedures. Non-indicated diagnostic testing increases the cost of care, may increase the risk of injury to the child, does not improve the outcome for the patient, and may be the source for adverse events. For example, acute viral respiratory tract infections are among the most common infectious problems of childhood. Although the majority of these infections do not require medical attention and are self-limited in nature, worried parents commonly bring their children to the ED for evaluation. The reluctance to come to a clinical diagnosis of a viral illness in such a child may cause the patient to undergo a constellation of precautionary and unnecessary diagnostic tests and may also result in the prescribing of unneeded and potentially harmful medications.

Fever is one of the most common reasons prompting acute illness evaluations in doctor's offices and EDs. In 2006, it accounted for approximately 3.3 million ED visits for children in the U.S.[7] Fever has been associated with a broad range of illnesses, ranging from serious and potentially life-threatening infections, to minor viral illnesses. Viral illnesses are by far the most common cause of fever in all pediatric age groups. The decision to pursue diagnostic testing in well-appearing febrile children requires an understanding of the relative risk for these more serious causes. The risk for a serious bacterial infection is sufficiently high in the neonatal population, and in children with underlying disorders (or the treatment of those disorders) causing a state of immunodeficiency, such that routine diagnostic testing and even empiric treatment (e.g., antibiotics) may be warranted.

Whether this same empiric testing approach should be applied to well-appearing febrile children without well-accepted risk factors for serious infections has been a subject of great interest and numerous studies in pediatric emergency care. Thanks to widespread immunization (which arguably has been the most important scientific achievement in pediatric care) the incidence of invasive disease from organisms such as H. influenzae and S. pneumoniae has been substantially reduced, and in the case of H. flu, nearly eliminated.[8] Although the risk for a potentially serious occult infection in a febrile well-appearing infant remains (particularly urinary infections), the practice of routine screening and empiric treatment for infections such as occult bacteremia in this population may in fact pose greater harm than good. Even in pediatric tertiary centers with presumably excellent technical skill, the risk of a falsely positive test, such as a contaminated blood culture, may be several times that of a true positive.[9] It also appears that the widespread practice of empiric therapy with potent broad-spectrum antibiotics has contributed to the rapid rise of multi-drug resistant organisms. As previously mentioned, emergency care providers need to be aware of demographic and clinical factors that pose additional risk for serious illness or injury for key presenting symptoms, and the differences in disease prevalence within each pediatric age group.

Another factor influencing utilization of diagnostic studies in children is the presence of a language barrier. One study found significant differences in test-ordering behavior and length of stay when physicians perceived the presence of a language barrier with patients.[10] Controlling for multiple other demographic and clinical factors, the study reported mean test charges were significantly higher and patients remained in the ED an average of 20 minutes longer when a language barrier was present. A possible explanation is that physicians were compensating for the diminished diagnostic power of the medical interview by increasing the intensity of laboratory and radiographic investigations. Providers may also have believed that patients with language barriers, independent of socioeconomic factors, were less likely to understand and comply with follow-up instructions. Therefore, an increased degree of assurance regarding the child's condition before discharge was required.[10]

Unnecessary diagnostic and therapeutic interventions can lead to prolonged ED length of stay, which may contribute to care quality and safety concerns in a busy ED. Although much progress has been made in the management of pain and anxiety, these interventions are typically painful and frightening for a child and can lead to adverse patient events, particularly related to the administration of medications. In contributing to the ED's potential to become a choke point in an organization, where a slowed delivery of care impacts the flow of care in other departments, these interventions can also result in significant direct and indirect costs to the health care system, as well as time lost to the children and their families, including missed school for the child and missed work for the parents. Sidebar 6-2, page 104, offers tips for addressing a parent's request for unnecessary medications and diagnostics.

Addressing Parents' Requests for Unnecessary Medication and Diagnostics

Understandably, some parents enter the ED in an anxious and concerned state when their child is experiencing a medical emergency, and they may have preconceived expectations of what their child needs from the ED staff, including medications, tests, procedures, or being admitted to the hospital. When these expectations are not met, these parents may become more persistent about their concerns. ED staff should remember to:

- Be patient and listen to their concerns.

- Be sensitive to their suggestions and knowledge about their child's condition. This is especially important when caring for children with special health care needs.

- Answer their questions when possible.

- When answers to questions are not available, tell them that you or another health care professional will share information with them when it becomes available.

- Allay fears when certain tests are or are not performed. Explain that there are other implications put upon children when unnecessary tests are conducted.

- Employ the assistance of the child's primary care physician in explaining the rationale for the care provided.

- Do not become defensive.

Source: Frush, Karen B.S.N., M.D. Chief Patient Safety Officer, Duke University Health System. Telephone interview on June 15, 2007.

Developing Emergency Care Practices That Involve Patient Families

ED care providers encounter families at a highly stressful time; there may be nothing more terrifying for a parent than the presence of a serious injury or illness. It is natural for a parent to believe his or her child is in desperate need of care, even when the clinician's assessment of severity is different. However, this can lead to a parent misinterpreting a child's symptoms and incorporating them into a child's history or the request of medically unnecessary diagnostic tests or medications.

It is important that ED clinicians possess the professional skills necessary to deliver care in a way that addresses parents' concerns and that parents are involved in all aspects of the care process. Whenever possible, ED clinicians should attempt to gain as much information as possible from the pediatric patient. Parents are typically a valuable (and frequently, the only) source for information and can be quite helpful in various components of care, providing emotional support for their children, and holding and/or assisting with diagnostic and therapeutic procedures.

As discussed in Chapter 3, a family-centered approach to care revolves around collaborating with parents or guardians and keeping them informed about the child's condition, prognosis, and treatment. In encouraging their involvement, even permitting them to be present during invasive procedures as long as the safety of the patient and medical providers is not compromised, clinicians can reduce or eliminate patient and family anxiety and combativeness as well as liability issues if parents or guardians are involved in decision making.

Assessing the Risks and Benefits of Medical Imaging for Children

Advancements in diagnostic testing, particularly in medical imaging, have contributed significantly to modern emergency care. One of the most notable has been computerized tomography (CT), which is nearly universally available for ED care providers and present in even the smallest hospitals. Over the past decade, CT has become increasingly pediatric-friendly, with faster scanning technology eliminating the need for sedation for the majority of patients.

Studies have demonstrated a remarkable growth in CT utilization, by as much as 600% since the mid-1980s.[11] It is estimated that 60 million CT studies are obtained annually in the United States, with an estimated annual utilization in children ranging from 4 to 7 million.[12–14] This rapid growth in utilization has been driven by the increased availability of CT, but other factors have also contributed. Requests by referring physicians, patient and family expectations, emergency care provider concerns for liability risk, and efforts to improve patient throughput in increasingly overcrowded EDs have all contributed to this growth.[11] These same factors have resulted in increased utilization of other diagnostic imaging modalities.

There is growing concern within radiology and other professional organizations that the ionizing radiation imparted by medical imaging, and particularly CT, which results in a radiation dose equivalent to approximately 150 to 250 chest x-rays (*see* Table 6-5), may pose a significant lifetime risk for the development of cancer in children.[12–17] Adult patients are also at risk, but it has been suggested that the risk is substantially greater in children for the following reasons:

- For the most part, tissues and organs that are growing and developing are more sensitive to radiation effects than those that are fully mature. It has been estimated that children may be 10 times more radiosensitive than adults.

- The oncogenic effect of radiation may have a long (for example, decades) latent period. This latent period varies with the type of malignancy. Leukemia has a shorter latency period (approximately 10 years) than solid malignancies. An infant or child has a much longer life expectancy in which to manifest the potential oncogenic effects of radiation compared with older adults.

- In the case of CT scanning, the radiation exposure from a fixed set of CT parameters results in a dose that is relatively higher for a child's smaller cross-sectional area compared with an adult.[13]

Cancer risk estimates, which represent extrapolations from studies of the survivors of the Hiroshima atomic bomb explosion, range anywhere from 1:1000 to 1:3000 for a CT scan.[15-17] It has been estimated that 1% to 2% of all cancer in the United States today is attributable to medical imaging.[12] The risk for cancer may be especially great for the youngest and most medically complex pediatric patients, who are subjected to a disproportionate amount of imaging studies.

ED clinicians play a central role in the use of CT in children, which includes making the decision when a CT scan is necessary and discussing the relative benefits and risks with patients and families. Recent studies indicate that patient families will welcome discussions regarding the relative risks and benefits of diagnostic and therapeutic interventions, including medical imaging.[18] Once informed, they may accept alternative modalities, such as observation over imaging. Informing patients and their families and partnering with them in medical decision-making are fundamental principles of patient- and family-centered care and will add significantly to efforts to improve patient safety.[19–21]

When the indications are clear, however, there is wide agreement that the benefits of a CT scan (and likewise, other medically indicated imaging studies) far outweigh the risks. Families and patients should be encouraged to

TABLE 6-5

Estimated Medical Radiation Doses for a 5-Year-Old Child

Imaging Modality and Area	Effective Dose, mSv	Equivalent Number of Two View Chest X-rays
3-view ankle	0.0015	1/14th
2-view chest	0.02	1
Anteroposterior and lateral abdomen	0.05	2
Tc-99m[2] radionuclide cystogram	0.18	9
Tc-99m radionuclide bone scan	6.2	310
FDG PET[3] scan	15.3	765
Fluoroscopic cystogram	0.33	16
Head CT	4	200
Chest CT	3	150
Abdomen CT	6	250

Tc-99m, technetium 99m; FDG PET, fluorodeoxyglucose positron emission tomography; mSv, millisievert.

Brody A.S., Frush D.P., Huda W., Brent R.L.: Section on Radiology: Radiation risk to children from computed tomography. Clinical report. *Pediatrics* 120:677–682, 2007. Printed with permission.

ask questions about the risks and benefits of CT and other imaging, and radiologists and pediatric medical and surgical sub-specialists (e.g., neurosurgeons, orthopedic surgeons) should be consulted when forming imaging strategies. It is also crucial for ED care providers to become familiar with the imaging practices within their hospital and, through collaboration with clinical leadership of the radiology department, assure that imaging equipment and protocols support reduced exposures (e.g., as low as reasonably achievable [ALARA]) for children. The need for those discussions is supported by literature suggesting that the imaging practice in many hospitals that perform CT imaging on children may not include appropriate dose adjustments.[22] This pediatric patient-specific approach should be applied to all ED clinical practices and all diagnostic resources that would be utilized in caring for children. The principles of the Image Gently Campaign, developed by the Alliance for Radiation Safety in Pediatric Imaging, a 13-member organization that includes leading medical professional societies and regulatory agencies, provide guidance on safe imaging practices that should be embraced by all health care facilities serving children[23]:

- Reduce or child-size the amount of radiation used.

- Scan only when necessary.

- Scan only the indicated region.

- Scan once; Multi-phase scanning is usually not necessary in children.

ED clinicians should also make a commitment to maintain awareness of published research that may elucidate clinical decision rules, risk factors, and other evidence that may assist in determining which children may be safely cared for without utilizing diagnostic studies that impart high doses of ioning radiation, and likewise, which children or injury patterns that merit these studies.

Being Prepared for Pediatric Trauma

Recognizing and responding to the anatomic, physiologic, and developmental differences of pediatric patients is never more important than when a seriously injured child arrives in the ED. In 2002, more than 6.8 million children ages 14 and under were injured, including more than 200,000 victims of violence.[24] Injury results in more deaths in children and adolescents than all other causes combined, accounting for 59.5% of all deaths in children younger than 18 years of age in 2004.[25] Trauma is also the leading cause of permanent disability in children.[26] Overall, it is estimated that 25% of children sustain an unintentional injury requiring medical care each year.[27] Improving outcomes for injured children requires the recognition of trauma as a significant public health problem. Efforts should be made to improve prehospital and hospital-based emergency medical care, trauma systems, and injury prevention programs for pediatric patients.[25]

Even in regions with well-developed trauma systems and designated care centers, most injured children are treated in hospitals without a trauma center designation.[28,29] Hospital and trauma system administrators should recognize that all hospital EDs may be required to evaluate and resuscitate

injured children.[25,30–32] Optimal preparation of the ED may be achieved through the designation of physician and nursing coordinators for pediatric emergency care, which is recommended in the 2006 IOM report and by the AAP, ACEP, and ENA in their joint pediatric preparedness guidelines.[1,3] All EDs should have protocols for the triage, treatment (within the scope of services available at the hospital), and transfer of injured children.

When a regional pediatric referral center is available, the most severely injured children often are eventually transported to that facility.[28] It has been shown that younger and more seriously injured children have better outcomes at a trauma center within a children's hospital or at a trauma center that integrates pediatric and adult trauma services.[28,33–36] The ability to provide a broad range of pediatric subspecialty services, including the presence of physicians trained in pediatric emergency care, pediatric critical care, pediatric surgical specialists, pediatric anesthesiologists, and pediatric medical subspecialists, is important. A pediatric intensive care unit staffed by health care professionals with appropriate training and experience in the care of the critically ill child is essential. Rehabilitation is another key component of optimal pediatric trauma care. Returning the injured child to full, age-appropriate function with the ability to reach his or her maximum potential is the ultimate goal. Sidebar 6-3, page 107, provides a series of recommendations from the AAP's 2008 policy statement on trauma systems and pediatric trauma care.[25]

Anticipating the Interfacility Transfer of Pediatric Patients

Recognizing that seriously injured or ill children may present to any ED, all hospitals must be prepared to effectively assess and provide appropriate initial stabilization for these patients, including those with ready access to local or regional pediatric tertiary care centers. Anticipating that the needs of certain pediatric patients may exceed the definitive care capabilities of the hospital, the ED should have a well-defined process for the interfacility transfer of children who require a higher level of care. Procedures for the interfacility transfer of patients should include the following components and pediatric patient considerations[3]:

1. Defined process for initiation of transfer, including the roles and responsibilities of the referring facility and referral center (including responsibilities for requesting transfer and communication).

2. Transport plan to deliver children safely and in a timely manner to the appropriate facility capable of providing definitive care.

| Sidebar 6-3 | **Recommendations for Pediatric Trauma Care** |

- The unique needs of injured children need to be integrated specifically into trauma systems and emergency and disaster planning in every state and region.

  - Pediatric surgical specialists and pediatric medical subspecialists should participate at all levels of planning for trauma, emergency, and disaster care.

- Every state should identify appropriate facilities with the resources to care for injured children and establish continuous monitoring processes for care delivered to injured children. Ensuring that the appropriate resources are available is especially important for the youngest and most severely injured children.

- All potential providers of pediatric emergency and trauma care should be familiar with their regional trauma system and be able to evaluate, stabilize, and transfer acutely injured children.

  - Although qualified pediatric critical care transport teams should be used when available in the interfacility transport of critically injured children, evaluation and management should begin with the care providers at the first point of entry into the trauma system.

- Every pediatric and emergency care-related health professional credentialing and certification body should define pediatric emergency and trauma care competencies and require practitioners to receive the appropriate level of initial and continuing education to achieve and maintain those competencies.

- Efforts to define and maintain pediatric care competencies should target both out-of-hospital and hospital-based care providers.

- Evidence-based protocols for management of the injured child should be developed for every aspect of care, from prehospital to postdischarge.

- Research, including data collection for best practices in isolated trauma and mass-casualty events, should be supported.

- Pediatric injury management should include an integrated public health approach, from prevention through prehospital care, to emergency and acute hospital care, to rehabilitation and long-term follow-up.

- National organizations with a special interest in pediatric trauma should collaborate to advocate for a higher and more consistent quality of care within the nation.

- National organizations with a special interest in pediatric trauma should collaborate to advocate for injury-prevention research and application of known prevention strategies into practice.

- State and federal financial support for trauma system development and maintenance must be provided.

- Steps should be taken to increase the number of trainees in specialties that care for injured children to address key subspecialty service shortages in pediatric trauma care. Strategies should include increased funding for graduate medical education and appropriate reimbursement for trauma specialists.

American Academy of Pediatrics Section on Orthopaedics, Committee on Pediatric Emergency Medicine, Section on Critical Care, Section on Surgery, Section on Transport Medicine, Committee on Pediatric Emergency Medicine, Pediatric Orthopaedic Society Of North America: Management of pediatric trauma. *Pediatrics* 121(4):849–854, 2008. Printed with permission.

3. Process for selecting the appropriate care facility for pediatric specialty services not available at the hospital. These specialty services may include:

   a. Medical and surgical specialty care.

   b. Critical care.

   c. Reimplantation (replacement of severed digits or limbs).

   d. Trauma and burn care.

   e. Psychiatric emergencies.

   f. Obstetric and perinatal emergencies.

   g. Child maltreatment (physical and sexual abuse and assault).

   h. Rehabilitation for recovery from critical medical or traumatic conditions.

4. Process for selecting the appropriately staffed transport service to match the patient's acuity level (e.g., level of care required by patient, equipment needed in transport) and appropriate for children with special health care needs.

5. Process for patient transfer (including obtaining informed consent).

6. Plan for transfer of patient information (e.g., medical record and copy of signed transport consent), personal belongings of the patient, and provision of directions and referral institution information to family.

7. Process for return transfer of the pediatric patient to the referring facility as appropriate.

As the interfacility transfer of a critically ill child may be a fairly infrequent event, the transfer process may be facilitated by the presence of a written policy and checklist to guide the staff, and to assure that all necessary steps are taken, and to assure compliance with Emergency Medical Treatment and Active Labor Act requirements.[37] The proactive development of a pediatric transfer agreement and the identification of a neonatal and pediatric critical care transport provider will reduce uncertainty and save precious time. Considering the growing prevalence of ED overcrowding and critical care bed shortages in pediatric tertiary centers, plans should also consider alternate care providers for those situations when the usual transport care provider and/or the preferred receiving hospital are unable to provide care.

Maintaining Vigilance for Non-Accidental Trauma and Child Maltreatment

ED staff must be aware of sentinel signs and maintain a level of vigilance for non-accidental trauma and other forms of child maltreatment. Child maltreatment is defined as harm resulting from inappropriate child-rearing practices.[38] Maltreatment manifests via several mechanisms, including physical abuse,[39] sexual abuse,[40] emotional abuse,[41] neglect,[42] and Munchausen's Syndrome by Proxy.[43] Neglect accounts for more than 60% of all maltreatment cases and parents are the perpetrators of maltreatment nearly 80% of the time. Sadly, this is a relatively common problem affecting children and families, and abuse and neglect are a significant cause of pediatric morbidity and mortality.[38]

According to the Administration for Children and Families, there were an estimated 3.3 million referrals to Child Protective Services agencies involving the alleged maltreatment of almost 6 million children.[44] For every case reported, it is estimated that another two cases go unrecognized. An estimated 900,000 children were deemed to be a victim of abuse or neglect during 2006.[44] Infants had the highest rate of victimization (24.4 per 1,000 children), approximately twice the rate for all children combined.[44] As previously mentioned, maltreatment is a leading cause of mortality, resulting in an estimated 1,530 deaths during 2006.[44]

Although certain patients and families may bear an increased risk for maltreatment, particularly children with disabilities,[45] physical abuse involves all segments of the population. Early detection and intervention may help to prevent future and potentially more severe or lethal assaults. In providing care for an injured child, ED clinicians should look for the following red flags that could suggest abuse:

- Patterned injuries, such as cigarette burns, rope burns, belt marks, or bite marks

- Atypical bruising locations (abdomen, chest, back, buttocks, ear, or neck) or number of bruises (e.g., more than 10 bruises) or bruising in infants that are not yet mobile (e.g., not yet "cruising")

- Multiple fractures in various stages of healing or fracture in the absence of reported trauma, or fractures of any kind in children less than one year of age without a clear and confirmed cause of injury

- Retinal hemorrhage or subdural bleeding

- Genital bleeding, lacerations, or infections

- History of unexplained or repeated injuries

- Discrepancies between the parents' explanation of how the injury occurred and the physical findings

- Developmental inability of the child to perform the action that parents say caused injury

- Delay in seeking treatment or travel to an ED far from the site of the accident or injury

- Inability on the part of the parents or caregiver to provide a history for the presenting complaint (e.g., limb disuse) or the suspicion that the history has been fabricated

- Frequent visits to various providers and EDs. Parents avoid going to the same hospital so patterns won't be identified

Bruises are obviously a common occurrence in childhood yet are also by far the most common sign of physical abuse.[46] When a child with external signs of trauma, such as bruising or one or more fractures, presents to the ED, differentiating accidental versus non-accidental trauma requires an awareness of common injury mechanism and knowledge of the developmental capabilities of the child.[47,48] ED staff must also maintain an appreciation for symptoms and signs (e.g., vomiting, irritability), particularly in infants and preverbal children, that could represent occult trauma. Table 6-6 provides a list of injuries, signs, or symptoms where non-accidental or inflicted trauma should be included in the differential diagnosis of children *less than four years of age*.[49] Staff should take care to accurately

TABLE 6-6

Injuries, signs, or symptoms where inflicted trauma/physical abuse is included in the differential diagnosis in children < 4 years of age

1. Musculoskeletal
a. any fracture in a child age <1 year and/or non-ambulating
b. any fracture in a child age <4 years without a plausible explanation
c. more than one fracture
d. abuse-concerning fractures: CML, rib, complex skull
e. high-energy fractures not accounted for by mechanism in history; transverse, comminuted, multiple, pelvic, scapular, sternal
f. delay in seeking care and fracture type is NOT buckle or hairline
g. unexplained limb disuse or swelling

2. Skin
a. any bruise in a non-ambulating child
b. any bruise in an abuse-concerning location such as: ear, frenulum, neck, chest, abdomen, back, buttocks, or GU
c. >4 bruises (excluding shins) in the ambulating child
d. any patterned bruising
e. history of "easy bruising" in an infant

3. Brain
a. any ICH in a child age <1 and/or non-ambulating
b. any ICH in a child age <4 without plausible explanation
c. full or bulging fontanel in the infant
d. unexplained seizure, headache, or ataxia
e. vomiting without diarrhea or fever in the child <4 years of age

4. Abdomen
a. abdominal wall bruising in a child <4 years without a plausible explanation
b. solid organ injury in a child age <4 years without a plausible explanation
c. duodenal hematoma in a child age <4 years without a plausible explanation
d. unexplained pancreatitis in a child age <4 years
e. bilious vomiting in a child age <4 years

5. Infant: signs and symptoms of inflicted trauma commonly misidentified
a. vomiting without diarrhea or fever
b. colic/fussy/irritable
c. apnea/ALTE spells
d. seizure

Abbreviations: CML, classic metaphyseal lesion; GU, genitourinary; ICH, intracranial hemorrhage; ALTE, apparent life threatening event.

Pierce M.C.: Appendix 1. Injuries, signs, or symptoms where inflicted trauma/physical abuse is included in the differential diagnosis in children < 4 years of age. *Clin Pediatr Emerg Med* 7:200, 2006. Reprinted with permission.

document conversations and findings in the patient medical record, ensuring that the information is available for the entire health care team and child family services.

All ED care providers should be prepared to consider and address the possibility of child maltreatment when there is reasonable cause for suspicion. The evaluation of the reported child sexual abuse victim is further complicated by the frequent absence of overt clinical findings.[50] Of course, not every ED may have the expertise or resources on-site to complete all components of the necessary evaluation. Specialized child protection resources may be available to

the ED on a consultative basis or may require that the patient be transferred to another facility for access to those services and an acute evaluation. The National Association of Children's Hospitals and Related Institutions has recently published guidelines for the establishment and management of hospital-based child protection teams.[51] Clinical policies or decision tools may prove to be useful in guiding ED staff in the difficult decision as to when it is appropriate to report physical or sexual abuse (*see* Table 6-7, page 110).[40] Clinical guidelines can also be a valuable resource regarding current best practices for diagnostic studies that should be performed on-site (e.g., which imaging or laboratory

TABLE 6-7

Guidelines for Making the Decision to Report Sexual Abuse in Children

Data Available				Response	
History	Behavioral Symptoms	Physical Examination	Diagnostic Tests	Level of Concern About Sexual Abuse	Report Decision
Clear statement	Present or absent	Normal or abnormal	Positive or negative	High	Report
None or vague	Present or absent	Normal or nonspecific	Positive test for C trachomatis, gonorrhea, T vaginalis, HIV, syphilis, or herpes*		
None or vague	Present or absent	Concerning or diagnostic findings	Negative or positive	High†	Report
Vague, or history by parent only	Present or absent	Normal or nonspecific	Negative	Indeterminate	Refer when possible
None	Present	Normal or nonspecific	Negative	Indeterminate	Possible report,‡ refer, or follow

* If nonsexual transmission is unlikely or excluded.
† Confirmed with various examination techniques and/or peer review with expert consultant.
‡ If behaviors are rare/unusual in normal children.

Source: Kellogg N.D., American Academy of Pediatrics Committee on Child Abuse and Neglect: The evaluation of sexual abuse in children. Clinical report. *Pediatrics* 116:506–512, 2005. Printed with permission.

studies to obtain),[52] documentation expectations, and which patients require referral for emergent evidentiary examinations versus those that can be referred for ambulatory follow-up. Checklists may be useful in assuring that all necessary steps are completed.

It is essential for ED clinical staff to be familiar with hospital policies and local reporting requirements for suspected child maltreatment. All 50 states and the District of Columbia have laws that require health care providers to report suspected cases of child abuse to the appropriate authority, typically a state or local social services, health department, or law enforcement agency. These same mandatory reporting statutes offer legal protection to reporters. Failure to report suspected maltreatment may not only expose the patient (or the parent in the case of intimate partner violence) to additional abusive injury but may also pose legal risk for the hospital and ED care providers. Legal concerns aside, considering the likely presence of significant physical and psychological harm to the patient, and the potential for continued abuse and the associated morbidity and mortality risks, ED staff must maintain a level of competency in their surveillance for maltreatment. In addition to the clinical reports and review articles cited in this chapter, there are numerous textbooks, journals, and web-based education resources available to assist in efforts to promote continuing professional education in this area.[53–56]

Mental Health Emergencies in Children and Adolescents

EDs play a vital role in the evaluation and management of children and adolescents with mental health emergencies.[57] According to the U.S. Surgeon General, 21% of children between the ages of 9 and 17 have a diagnosable mental health disorder.[58] Mental health emergencies constitute a growing segment of pediatric emergency medical care. Nationwide, hospitals have reported substantial increases in visits made by pediatric patients seeking mental health services, with reported increases over the past decade ranging from 100 to 600 percent.[59–62] Mental health related diagnoses constituted approximately 5% of all ED visits made by children in the United States from 1995–2001.[61]

There are many reasons for this profound increase in ED utilization by children and families.[62] Community-based ambulatory and inpatient mental health resources have diminished, and in some regions, even disappeared. Critical shortages of both inpatient beds and pediatric-trained mental health specialists exist in most communities.[63] Access to limited local resources may be especially challenging for the uninsured and those with public health insurance. Only 20% of children who need mental health services receive them.[58] The ED has increasingly become the safety net for children and adolescents, with mental health disorders that are not addressed by a fragmented mental health care delivery system.[57]

TABLE 6-8

Depressive Symptoms and Examples in Adolescents

Signs and Symptoms of Major Depressive Disorder	Signs of Depression Frequently Seen in Youth
Depressed mood most of the day	Irritable or cranky mood; preoccupation with song lyrics that suggest life is meaningless
Decreased interest/enjoyment in once favorite activities	Loss of interest in sports, video games, and activities with friends
Significant weight loss/gain	Failure to gain weight as normally expected; anorexia or bulimia; frequent complaints of physical illness; eg, headache, stomach ache
Insomnia or hypersomnia	Excessive late-night TV; refusal to wake for school in the morning
Psychomotor agitation/retardation	Talk of running away from home, or efforts to do so
Fatigue or loss of energy	Persistant boredom
Low self-esteem; feelings of guilt	Oppositional and/or negative behavior
Decreased ability to concentrate; indecisive	Poor performance in school; frequent absences
Recurrent suicidal ideation or behavior	Recurrent suicidal ideation or behavior (writing about death; giving away favorite toys or belongings)

Reprinted with permission from the *Diagnostic and Statistical Manual of Mental Disorders*. Washington, D.C.: American Psychiatric Association; 2000.

This essential safety net role requires that emergency care professionals be aware of the prevalence and types of mental health disorders in children. In addition, they must be capable of performing an appropriate history and screening examination and be able to identify the presence of a mental health crisis. Based on the urgency and severity of the presenting concern and the degree of stress within the family unit, ED care providers must also be prepared to engage acute interventions, arrange psychiatric consultation, and plan disposition.[64] In addition to caring for children with mental retardation, autistic spectrum disorders, or those who are having a behavioral crisis, ED staff must also be capable of managing children with exacerbations of previously diagnosed mental illnesses.[57] They also must be prepared to identify and initiate care for patients with previously undiagnosed disorders such as suicidal ideation, depression, escalating aggression, substance abuse, and posttraumatic stress disorder.[57] ED staff must also evaluate victims of physical and sexual abuse, children exposed to community and domestic violence, and deal with unexpected deaths of children in the ED.[57, 65]

Mental health disorders in children are frequently not recognized as such, as they may initially present as somatic complaints, or trauma, and therefore can be overlooked. Children presenting to the ED may not be accompanied by a caregiver who can provide sufficient historical data to support the diagnosis. The presence of overcrowding may not always allow sufficient time to uncover mental health concerns as these patients typically require time and resource intensive assessments. In an ideal setting, pediatric mental health emergencies are best managed with a multidisciplinary team, utilizing specialized screening tools, pediatric-trained mental health consultants, the availability of pediatric psychiatric inpatient facilities when hospitalization is necessary, and an ambulatory care infrastructure that supports pediatric mental health care, including communication back to the child's medical home and timely and appropriate referrals to mental health professionals.[57]

Mental health disorders are also a significant cause of mortality in children. Suicide is the third leading cause of death for teenagers and the rate of suicide among adolescents in the United States has tripled since the 1950s.[66,67] As many

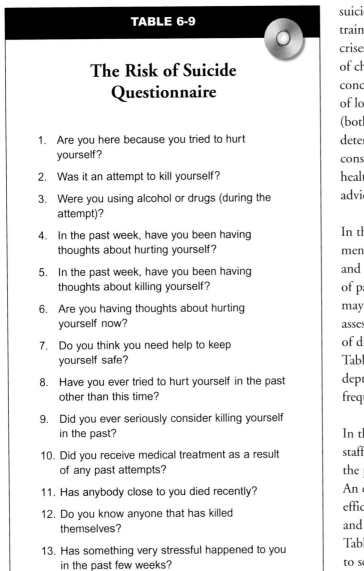

TABLE 6-9

The Risk of Suicide Questionnaire

1. Are you here because you tried to hurt yourself?

2. Was it an attempt to kill yourself?

3. Were you using alcohol or drugs (during the attempt)?

4. In the past week, have you been having thoughts about hurting yourself?

5. In the past week, have you been having thoughts about killing yourself?

6. Are you having thoughts about hurting yourself now?

7. Do you think you need help to keep yourself safe?

8. Have you ever tried to hurt yourself in the past other than this time?

9. Did you ever seriously consider killing yourself in the past?

10. Did you receive medical treatment as a result of any past attempts?

11. Has anybody close to you died recently?

12. Do you know anyone that has killed themselves?

13. Has something very stressful happened to you in the past few weeks?

14. Do you use alcohol or drugs?

Source: Horowitz L.M., Wang P.S., Koocher G.P., et al.: Detecting suicide risk in a pediatric emergency department: development of a brief screening tool. *Pediatrics* 2001; 107(5):1133–1137. Printed with permission.

as 12% of children ages 6 to 12 and 53% of adolescents age 13 to 19 have suicidal thoughts, and 250,000 adolescents attempt suicide each year. In 1997, the Centers for Disease Control Youth Risk Behavior Surveillance System reported that 21% of high school students had seriously considered attempting suicide, 16% had made a plan to attempt suicide, and nearly 8% had made an actual suicide attempt.[68]

The ED is often the first point of contact with the health care system for suicide attempters and adolescents with suicidal ideation. Despite the importance of recognizing suicidality in the ED setting, providers with specialized training in the recognition and management of psychiatric crises are often not immediately available. The presentation of children and adolescents with urgent mental health concerns must be anticipated, and identity and location of local and/or regional pediatric mental health services (both outpatient and inpatient) should be prospectively determined. In the absence of on-site ED psychiatry consultative services, support for the evaluation of mental health concerns by ED staff may be provided by telephonic advice.

In the absence of mental health specialty care support, non-mental health clinicians bear the responsibility for detecting and acutely managing mental health problems. The presence of patient care guidelines and other clinical decision-tools may prove to be useful in guiding ED clinicians in the assessment of mental health concerns, and in the detection of disorders, such as depression, in the pediatric population. Table 6-8 lists the typical symptoms and signs of a major depressive disorder and provides examples of signs frequently seen in youth.[67]

In the absence of on-site services to advise or assist ED staff in their assessment of high-risk mental health concerns, the presence of screening tools may prove to be life-saving. An effective screening instrument must be accurate, efficient, and acceptable (to both the provider and patient), and it must also be linked to an effective intervention.[60] Table 6-9 provides an example of a survey tool developed to screen pediatric ED patients for risk of suicide. This 14-item survey tool, the Risk for Suicide Questionnaire, which was specifically designed for use by non-mental health care professionals, accurately screens for the presence of suicide risk.[69]

In addition to this survey's accuracy and the brief time it takes to administer, there are other features of this brief screening tool that make it advantageous in ED settings. Evaluations of suicidality may be particularly stressful or avoided by clinicians who lack formal mental health training, do not have confidence in their psychological assessment and intervention skills, or are often uncomfortable treating this patient population. However, with proper structured tools to guide them, non-mental health clinicians can increase their confidence and lower barriers to asking about suicidal risk. In this study, nurses reported that having the screening tool was much preferred to the previous method of judging by intuition when and how to ask about suicidal behavior.[69]

In collaboration with pediatricians, mental health specialists, social workers, and child life specialists, ED leadership should develop policies and procedures that address all aspects of care for children and adolescents with mental health complaints. One very important topic is the use of physical and chemical restraints and alternative techniques (e.g., calming maneuvers, therapeutic holding, show of force, distraction) to consider. The need to restrain children and adolescents is uncommon and should occur only when pediatric patients pose harm to themselves or others. It is important that organizations develop precise written policies for restraint use that are guided by national standards and recommendations. As previously mentioned, ED staff will require policies providing guidance regarding available pediatric mental health resources and processes to access these specialized services. ED policies and practices must also recognize the primary support role of the family and caregivers in all phases of care for pediatric mental illness.

Adopting an Evidence-Based Approach to Pediatric Emergency Care

As physicians are being called on to justify their treatment decisions with valid, up-to-date evidence, the term "evidence-based medicine" has become a common health care catch phrase. There have been attempts within many areas of medicine to quantify the evidence that is available to, and used by, the physicians of that discipline. Although the Institute of Medicine and others have noted the need for more clinical research to support a more robust evidence base for emergency care practices,[1] and particularly for pediatric care, there is a growing foundation of clinical evidence to guide professionals as they care for children.

Within pediatrics, a small number of studies have searched for the presence of medical evidence to support clinical interventions. One study examining pediatric inpatient care found that 75% of primary interventions were supported by evidence.[70] Another study examining care provided in a community-based pediatric practice found that 40% of interventions were supported by evidence derived from a randomized control trial, and another 7% were supported by convincing non-experimental evidence.[71] A study of care provided in a pediatric ED found that only 12.5% of the interventions lacked level I (presence of a randomized controlled trial, systematic review, or meta-analysis) or II (presence of face validity in the absence of Level I evidence) supportive evidence.[72] Interestingly, 36% of the patients enrolled had no intervention at all in the ED. Although this study was conducted in a tertiary children's hospital ED, the findings are still relevant even in a community

hospital setting, as it demonstrates the presence of a reasonable evidence base to inform emergency professionals as they care for children.

More than a health care catch phrase, "evidence-based medicine" should be adopted in ED settings as part of every organization's commitment to delivering the highest quality of care to pediatric patients. Through continuing education and other activities intended to maintain pediatric care competencies, and by integrating an evidence-based approach to pediatric care, ED clinicians will be better able to recognize symptoms and signs of common and uncommon illnesses and diseases in children and intervene with appropriate diagnostic studies and effective therapeutic modalities.

References

1. Institute of Medicine, Committee on the Future of Emergency Care in the United States Health System: *Emergency care for children: growing pains.* Washington, D.C.: National Academies Press, 2006.

2. Gausche-Hill M., Schmitz C., Lewis R.J.: Pediatric preparedness of United States emergency departments: a 2003 survey. *Pediatrics* 120:1229–1237, 2007.

3. Gausche-Hill M., Krug S.E., and the American Academy of Pediatrics Committee on Pediatric Emergency Medicine, American College of Emergency Physicians Pediatric Committee, Emergency Nurses Association Pediatric Committee: Guidelines for care of children in the emergency department. *Pediatrics* 124: 1233–1243, Oct. 2009.

4. Gausche-Hill M., Fuchs S., Yamamoto L. (eds.), APLS: *The Pediatric Emergency Medicine Resource,* 4th ed. Sudbury, MA: Jones and Bartlett, 2004.

5. Dieckmann R. (ed.): *Pediatric Education for Prehospital Professionals,* 2nd ed. American Academy of Pediatrics. Sudbury, MA: Jones and Bartlett; 2005.

6. Ruddy R.M.: Abdominal pain. In Fleisher G.R., Ludwig S., Henretig F.M., Ruddy R., Silverman B.K. (eds.): *Textbook of Pediatric Emergency Medicine,* 5th ed. Philadelphia, PA: Lippincott, Williams & Wilkins, 2006, pp. 469–476.

7. Pitts S.R., Niska R.W., Xu J., Burt C.W.: National hospital ambulatory medical care survey: 2006 emergency department summary. National Health Statistics Reports, No. 7. Hyattsville, MD: National Center for Health Statistics, 2008.

8. American Academy of Pediatrics. Haemophilus influenza infections. In: Pickering L.K., Baker C.J., Long S.S., McMillan J.A. (eds.): *Red Book: 2006 Report of the Committee on Infectious Diseases.* 27th ed. Elk Grove Village, IL: American Academy of Pediatrics, 2006, pp. 310–318.

9. Alpern E.R., Alessandrini E.A., Bell L.M., Shaw K.N., et al.: Occult bacteremia from a pediatric emergency department: current prevalence, time to detection, and outcome. *Pediatrics* 106(3):505–511, 2000.

10. Hampers L.C., Susie Cha S., et al.: Language barriers and resource utilization in a pediatric emergency department. *Pediatrics* 103:1253–1256, 1999.

11. Krug S.E.: The art of communication: strategies to improve efficiency, quality of care and patient safety in the emergency department. *Pediatr Radiol* 38:S655–659, 2008.

12. Brenner D.J., Hall E.J.: Computed tomography—an increasing source of radiation exposure. *New Engl J Med* 357:2277–2284, 2007.

13. Brody A.S., Frush D.P., Huda W., Brent R.L.: Section on Pediatric Radiology: Radiation risk to children from computed tomography—Clinical report. *Pediatrics* 120:677–682, 2007.

14. Frush D.P., Donnelly L.F., Rosen N.S.: Computed tomography and radiation risks: what pediatric health care providers should know. *Pediatrics* 112:951–957, 2003.

15. Hall E.J.: Lessons we have learned from our children: cancer risks from diagnostic radiology. *Pediatr Radiol* 32:700–706, 2002.

16. Brenner D.J.: Estimating cancer risks from pediatric CT: going from the qualitative to the quantitative. *Pediatr Radiol* 32:228–231, 2002.

17. Brenner D.J., Elliston C.D., Hall E.J., Berdon W.E.: Estimated risks of radiation-induced fatal cancer from pediatric CT. *Am J Radiol* 176:289–296, 2001.

18. Larson D.B., Rader S.B., Forman H.P., Fenton L.Z.: Informing parents about CT radiation exposure in children: it's OK to tell them. *Am J Radiol* 189:271–275, 2007.

19. Frush K.S., Krug S.E., American Academy of Pediatrics Committee on Pediatric Emergency Medicine: Patient safety in the pediatric emergency care setting. *Pediatrics* 120:1367–1375, 2007.

20. O'Malley P., Brown K., Mace S.E., American Academy of Pediatrics Committee on Pediatric Emergency Medicine: Patient and family centered care and the role of the emergency physician in providing care to a child in the emergency department. *Pediatrics* 118:2242–2244, 2006.

21. Graedon J., Graedon T.: Enlisting families as patient safety allies. *Clin Pediatr Emerg Med* 7:265–267, 2006.

22. Patterson A., Frush D.P., Donnelly L.F.: Helical CT of the body: are settings adjusted for pediatric patients? *Am J Radiol* 176:297–301, 2001.

23. Goske M.J., Applegate K.E., Boylan J., et al.: The image gently campaign: working together to change practice. *Am J Radiol* 190:273–274, 2008. Available at: http://www.ajronline.org/cgi/content/full/190/2/273 (accessed Jul. 1, 2009).

24. Centers for Disease Control and Prevention, National Center for Injury Prevention and Control: "Web-based Injury Statistics Query and Reporting System (WISQARS)." March 5, 2004. Available at: www.cdc.gov/ncipc/wisqars (accessed Feb. 4, 2009).

25. Tuggle D., Krug S., American Academy of Pediatrics Section on Orthopaedics, Committee on Pediatric Emergency Medicine, Section on Critical Care, Section on Surgery, Section on Transport Medicine, Committee on Pediatric Emergency Medicine, Pediatric Orthopaedic Society Of North America: Management of pediatric trauma. *Pediatrics* 121(4):849–854, 2008.

26. Arias E., MacDorman M.F., Strobino D.M., Guyer B.: Annual summary of vital statistics. *Pediatrics* 112:1215–1230, 2003.

27. Danesco E.R., Miller T.R., Spicer R.S.: Incidence and costs of 1987–1994 childhood injuries: demographic breakdowns. *Pediatrics* 105(2):e27, 2000. Available at: www.pediatrics.org/cgi/content/full/105/2/e27 (accessed Feb. 3, 2009).

28. Densmore J.C., Lim H.J., Oldham K.T., Guice K.S.: Outcomes and delivery of care in pediatric injury. *J Pediatr Surg* 41:92–98, 2006.

29. Segui-Gomez M., Chang D.C., Paidas C.N., et al.: Pediatric trauma care: an overview of pediatric trauma systems and their practices in 18 U.S. states. *J Pediatr Surg* 38:1162–1169, 2003.

30. American Academy of Pediatrics, Committee on Pediatric Emergency Medicine, Committee on Medical Liability, Task Force on Terrorism: The pediatrician and disaster preparedness. *Pediatrics* 117:560–565, 2006.

31. Pyles L.A., Knapp J.F., American Academy of Pediatrics, Committee on Pediatric Emergency Medicine: Role of pediatricians in advocating life support training courses for parents and the public. *Pediatrics* 114(6):e761–765, 2004. Available at: www.pediatrics.org/cgi/content/full/114/6/e761 (accessed Feb. 3, 2009).

32. American Academy of Pediatrics, Committee on Pediatric Emergency Medicine, American College of Emergency Physicians, Pediatric Committee: Care of children in the emergency department: guidelines for preparedness. *Pediatrics* 107:777–781, 2001.

33. Stylianos S., Egorova N., Guice K.S., Arons R.R., Oldham K.T.: Variation in treatment of pediatric spleen injury at trauma centers verses nontrauma centers: a call for dissemination of American pediatric surgical association benchmarks and guidelines. *J Am Coll Surg* 202:247–251, 2006.

34. MacKenzie E.J., Rivara F.P., Jurkovich G.J., et al.: A national evaluation of the effect of trauma-center care on mortality. *N Engl J Med* 354:366–378, 2006.

35. Davis D.H., Localio A.R., Stafford P.W., Helfaer M.A., Durbin D.R.: Trends in operative management of pediatric splenic injury in a regional trauma system. *Pediatrics* 115:89–94, 2005.

36. Odetola F.O., Miller W.C., Davis M.M., Bratton S.L.: The relationship between the location of pediatric intensive care unit facilities and child death from trauma: a county level ecologic study. *J Pediatr* 147:74–77, 2005.

37. Teshome G., Closson F.T.: Emergency Medical Treatment and Labor Act: the basics and other medicolegal concerns. *Pediatr Clin North Am* 53(1):139–155, 2006.

38. Berkowitz C.D., Carroll M.L.: Child maltreatment. In Gausche-Hill M., Fuchs S.M., Yamamoto L. (eds.): APLS: *The Pediatric Emergency Resource,* 4th ed. Sudbury, MA: Jones and Bartlett, 2004, pp. 324–359.

39. Kellogg N.D., American Academy of Pediatrics Committee on Child Abuse and Neglect: Evaluation of suspected child physical abuse. Clinical report. *Pediatrics* 119(6):1232–1241, 2007.

40. Kellogg N.D., American Academy of Pediatrics Committee on Child Abuse and Neglect: The evaluation of sexual abuse in children. Clinical report. *Pediatrics* 116:506–512, 2005.

41. Kairys S.W., Johnson C.F., American Academy of Pediatrics Committee on Child Abuse and Neglect: The psychological maltreatment of children. Technical report. *Pediatrics* 109(4):e68, 2002. Available at: http://www.aap.org (accessed Feb. 4, 2009).

42. Jenny C., American Academy of Pediatrics Committee on Child Abuse and Neglect: Recognizing and responding to medical neglect. Clinical report. *Pediatrics* 120(6):1385–1389, 2007.

43. Stirling J., American Academy of Pediatrics Committee on Child Abuse and Neglect: Beyond Munchausen syndrome by proxy: identification and treatment of child abuse in a medical setting. Clinical report. *Pediatrics* 119(5):1026–1030, 2007.

44. Administration for Children and Families: Summary—Child Maltreatment 2006. U.S. Department of Health and Human Services. Available at: www.acf.hhs.gov/programs/cb/pubs/cm06/summary.htm (accessed Feb. 4, 2009).

45. Hibbard R.A., Desch L.W., American Academy of Pediatrics Committee on Child Abuse and Neglect, and Council on Children with Disabilities: Maltreatment of children with disabilities. *Pediatrics* 119:1018–1025, 2007.

46. Kaczor K., Pierce M.C., Makaroff K., Corey T.S.: Bruising and physical child abuse. *Clin Pediatr Emerg Med* 7:153–160, 2006.

47. Pierce M.C., Bertocci G.: Fractures resulting from inflicted trauma: assessing injury and history compatibility. *Clin Pediatr Emerg Med* 7:143–148, 2006.

48. Jenny C., American Academy of Pediatrics Committee on Child Abuse and Neglect: Evaluating infants and small children with multiple fractures. Clinical report. *Pediatrics* 118(3):1299–1003, 2006.

49. Pierce M.C.: Appendix 1. Injuries, signs, or symptoms where inflicted trauma/physical abuse is included in the differential diagnosis in children <4 years of age. *Clin Pediatr Emerg Med* 7:200, 2006.

50. Bernard D., Peters M., Makaroff K.: The evaluation of suspected pediatric sexual abuse. *Clin Pediatr Emerg Med* 7:161–169, 2006.

51. National Association of Children's Hospitals and Related Institutions: *Defining the children's hospital role in child maltreatment.* Alexandria, VA: National Association of Children's Hospitals and Related Institutions, 2006.

52. Pierce M.C.: Appendix 2. Physical child abuse workup for children 4 years of age and younger in the emergency department. *Clin Pediatr Emerg Med* 7:201, 2006.

53. Ludwig S.: Child abuse. In Fleisher G.R., Ludwig S., Henretig F.M., Ruddy R., Silverman B.K. (eds.): *Textbook of Pediatric Emergency Medicine,* 5th ed. Philadelphia, PA: Lippincott, Williams & Wilkins, 2006, pp. 1761–1802.

54. Reece R.M., Ludwig S. (eds.): *Child Abuse: Medical Diagnosis and Management,* 2nd ed. Philadelphia, PA: Lea & Febinger, 2001.

55. Lau K., Krase K., Morse R.H.: *Mandated Reporting of Child Abuse and Neglect: a Practical Guide for Social Workers.* New York, NY: Springer, 2008.

56. Makaroff K.L.: Appendix 4. Fifty very useful child abuse articles for pediatric emergency medicine physicians. *Clin Pediatr Emerg Med* 7:204–211, 2006.

57. Dolan M.A., Mace S.E., American Academy of Pediatrics Committee on Pediatric Emergency Medicine, American College of Emergency Physicians Pediatric Emergency Medicine Committee: Pediatric mental health emergencies in the emergency medical services system. *Pediatrics* 118(4):1064–1067, 2006.

58. U.S. Public Health Service. Report of the U.S. Surgeon General's Conference on Children's Mental Health: A National Action Agenda. Washington, D.C.: U.S. Department of Health and Human Services, 1999.

59. Cooper J.L., Masi R.: Child and youth emergency mental health care: a national problem. National Center for Children in Poverty, Mailman School of Public Health, Columbia University, 2007. Available at: http://www.nccp.org/publications/pub_750.htm (accessed Feb. 5, 2009).

60. Baren J.M., Mace S.E., Hendry P.L., et al.: Children's mental health emergencies—part 1: challenges in care: definition of the problem, barriers to care, screening, advocacy, and resources. *Pediatr Emerg Care* 24(6):399–408, 2008.

61. Grupp-Phelan J., Harman J.S., Kelleher K.J.: Trends in mental health and chronic conditions visits by children presenting for care at U.S. emergency departments. *Pub Health Rep* 122:55–61, 2007.

62. Edelsohn G.A. Urgency counts: the why behind pediatric psychiatric emergency visits. *Clin Pediatr Emerg Med* 5:146–153, 2004.

63. American Academy of Pediatrics Committee on Child Health Financing: Scope of health care benefits from birth through age 21. *Pediatrics* 117:979–982, 2006.

64. Baren J.M., Mace S.E., Hendry P.L., et al.: Children's mental health emergencies—part 2: emergency department evaluation and treatment of children with mental health disorders. *Pediatr Emerg Care* 24(7):485–498, 2008.

65. Baren J.M., Mace S.E., Hendry P.L., et al.: Children's mental health emergencies—part 3: special situations: child maltreatment, violence, and response to disasters. *Pediatr Emerg Care* 24(8):569–577, 2008.

66. Spirito A., Lewander W.: Assessment and disposition planning for adolescent suicide attempters treated in the emergency department. *Clin Pediatr Emerg Med* 5:154–163, 2004.

67. Shain B.N., American Academy of Pediatrics Committee on Adolescence: Suicide and suicide attempts in adolescents. Clinical report. *Pediatrics* 120(3):669–676, 2007.

68. Centers for Disease Control and Prevention: Youth-risk behavior surveillance, United States, 1997. *MMWR* 47:239–291, 1998.

69. Horowitz L., Wang P.S., Koocher G.P., et al.: Detecting suicide risk in a pediatric emergency department: development of a brief screening tool. *Pediatrics* 107(5)1133–1137, 2001.

70. Moyer V.A., Gist A.K., Elliot E.J.: Is the practice of paediatric inpatient medicine evidence-based? *Pediatr Child Health* 38:347–351, 2002.

71. Rudolf M.C., Lyth N., Bundle A., et al.: A search for the evidence supporting community paediatric practice. *Arch Dis Child;* 80:257–261, 1999.

72. Waters K.L., Wiebe N., Cramer K., et al.: Treatment in the pediatric emergency department is evidence based: a retrospective analysis. *BMC Pediatr* 6:26, 2006.

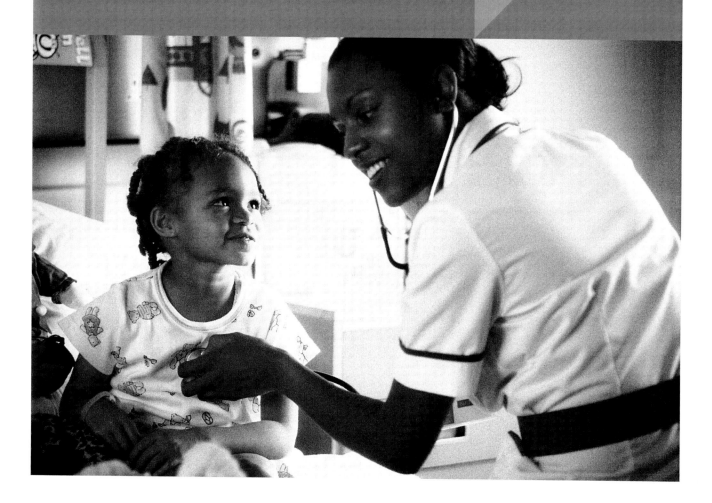

CHAPTER 7

Treating Children with Special Health Care Needs in the ED

Contributing Editor: Loren G. Yamamoto, M.D., M.P.H.,
Emergency Medicine Director and Vice Chief of Staff,
Kapi'olani Medical Center for Women and Children, Honolulu

"Special needs" children have or are at risk for chronic physical, developmental, behavioral, or emotional conditions and also require health and related services of a type or amount not usually required by typically developing children.[1] Special needs children often require emergency care for health maintenance, as well as acute life-threatening complications unique to their chronic conditions.

This chapter discusses the challenges that arise in treating these children in the ED while stressing the importance that clinicians be provided with access to their medical information at the outset of care. The chapter also presents some guidelines and references to other more comprehensive resources for the emergency care of children with special health care needs.

Understanding the Unique Issues in Caring for Children with Special Health Care Needs

As many as 9.4 million children—or 13% of United States children under the age of 18—are living with chronic medical conditions.[2] These special needs patients include children with cerebral palsy, spina bifida, asthma, cancer, hemophilia, autism, diabetes, congenital heart disease, as well as metabolic and genetic disorders. In all, about 20% of U.S. households with children have a special needs child.[2]

In addition to their increased risk for illness and morbidity from their chronic medical disorders, when children with special health care needs suffer an acute illness (such as an infection) or an injury, they are commonly at greater risk than other children for complications due to their underlying conditions.[2] Dependence on indwelling devices such as ventriculoperitoneal shunts, gastrostomy tubes, tracheostomy tubes, central vascular catheters, and congenital heart disease corrective/palliative devices place these patients at greater medical risk due to device failure, malfunction, or infection.

An added challenge of caring for children with special health care needs in an ED is that emergency care providers may not know or be informed about preexisting conditions, the potential for drug reactions and interactions, or the most optimal means of evaluating and treating recurrent health care needs of these patients, especially if ED providers are caring for such a patient for the first time.[2] Even children with easily recognized problems might be difficult to treat when a physician is unfamiliar with their medical history.[2] An example of this is latex allergy that is more common among certain special needs children. Although this is not a problem if these children are treated in latex-free facilities, an emergency encounter at a facility that is not latex-free will place these patients at significant risk for a potentially life-threatening reaction.

Advances in new and experimental therapeutic and diagnostic practices for children with special health care needs further challenge ED providers. A child's specialist may be the only one who knows about a new or experimental therapy and/or who is aware of an individualized treatment plan that took years to develop.[2] For example, a child with a rare metabolic disorder may require a specific type of feeding or IV infusion, and a child with cyanotic congenital heart disease and a dysrhythmia may require a specific medication regimen. Although some children with special health care needs have highly specialized and unique management requirements, many pediatric subspecialty conditions may be addressed through the creation and periodic updating of practice guidelines or clinical pathways for the expected manifestations of chronic disease (e.g., diabetic ketoacidosis, sickle cell crisis, asthma exacerbation, status epilepticus), acute illness concerns in high risk patients (e.g., fever in the immunosuppressed host), or for device-related problems (e.g., suspected ventriculoperitoneal shunt malfunction, tracheostomy tube occlusion, gastrostomy tube failure, etc.). These guidelines should be developed in consultation with the child's specialist and medical home. This advanced planning for the care of medically complex children can promote care consistency, patient safety, and may also save valuable time when these patients present acutely in the ED.

Ensuring Appropriate Emergency Information

Emergency care of children with special needs is frequently complicated by the absence of a comprehensive summary of their medical condition as well as the special precautions and therapeutic interventions to consider in the management of chronic disease or acute illness.[3] To address this issue, the American Academy of Pediatrics (AAP) and the American College of Emergency Physicians (ACEP) introduced a standardized emergency information form (EIF) for children with special health care needs that can be used to inform caregivers at all health care system levels of the child's medical conditions, medications, and treatment recommendations in an emergency.[3] Table 7-1, page 120, contains the AAP/ACEP standardized EIF. (*See* the CD for a sample EIF.) Health information summaries like the EIF should ultimately be revised to simplify the process of updating medical information and making changes, dating of these changes in the form (or data set) to support an assessment of whether it is up-to-date, ensuring access to this information, and facilitating the process of emergency care planning and disaster planning. Although this sounds like a reasonably simple task, this process is very time consuming and the implementation of an EIF system is complex because of compatibility problems with varying electronic medical record systems and ensuring accessibility under difficult circumstances (e.g., a disaster that could include infrastructure failure) while maintaining confidentiality. "Ideally, EIFs should be completed under the guidance of the pediatric practitioner in the patient's medical home," according to Francis E. Rushton, M.D. F.A.A.P., District IV Chair, American Academy of Pediatrics for Beaufort, "but the resources in many of today's practices are insufficient to meet this task. Of necessity, it should be a joint responsibility of the pediatric generalist, specialists and emergency room provider to ensure that the EIF is updated at each clinical encounter. Pediatric Electronic Health Records (EHRs) are currently evolving, and the definition of a 'meaningful use' standard is being discussed. A clear need from EHRs is the ability to abstract a useful up-to-date EIF at each visit to provide to the family of children with special health care needs."

The Minnesota Emergency Medical Services for Children program, in collaboration with the University of Minnesota Children's Hospital, the Children's Hospital of Minneapolis, and St. Paul Children's Hospital, and others, has developed a Web-based EIF access system known as MEMSCIS (Midwest Emergency Medical Services for Children Information System). MEMSCIS was initially piloted for a group of children with congenital heart disease, but has since grown to include more than 200 children with a variety of complex medical conditions. MEMSCIS offers secure on-line access to this information for parents and care providers. The system also provides a "break the glass" process for immediate access to the EIF in emergency situations.[4]

Encouraging an Emergency Care Plan for Children With Special Health Care Needs

The essential components of an emergency care plan should include a method for identifying special needs children, education of families, and the completion and updating of a health information data set such as the EIF by the child's primary or specialty care physicians and other health care professionals. Previous experience with the EIF for children with special health care needs has demonstrated difficulties with the completion and periodic updating of these forms.[3] It should also be noted that although maintenance of confidentiality and 24/7 rapid access to this information are both highly desirable, these two factors actually oppose each other. Thus, a realistic compromise must be made. Regulatory agencies, future legislation, and health care institutions must understand and accept this compromise as tightly secured patient confidentiality makes access to this vital information more difficult.

National organizations and government agencies, such as the U.S. Department of Health and Human Services, advocate the use of emergency data sets, summaries, or "passports," all of which are similar to EIFs.[3] In addition,

the Emergency Medical Services for Children (EMSC) program through its Children with Special Health Care Needs Task Force Report of January 1997, noted:

> "If the child is at risk for future medical emergencies, the child and family should participate in developing a written emergency care plan. Copies of this plan should be kept in easily accessible places at the child's home and any other location where the child regularly spends time. The plan should include provisions for any special training that will be needed by emergency medical personnel, family members, or other persons who may be called on to provide emergency care for the child."[5]

Standardizing an information system that accomplishes this would be desirable, with the understanding that different health care providers will require different levels of information for health maintenance versus what may be necessary to treat acute conditions. For example, the information needed by an ED would be different from that required by a school nurse. For a serious emergency, the care plan for the ED might include very specific medication orders, while the plan for a school nurse might be to call the parent or 911. Standardization is a complex issue because it includes standardizing data content, data format, methods of updating, storage devices, and the means of retrieving information. In reality, the combinations and permutations are exceedingly large, and it is unlikely that one standard will work for all parties involved; however, creating a standard with compatible alternatives would be a necessary first step to facilitate data access and interchange, while meeting the specific informational needs of patients and the different health care providers in various settings and levels of care.

Supportive elements of this strategy can include links to emergency services, such as 911, and window stickers identifying homes of children with special needs.[3] In theory, 911 systems can recognize phone numbers registered to a family with a special needs child (linkage to 911), which will alert emergency medical service (EMS) professionals to seek access to special health care needs information. Sophisticated online access could be obtained and communicated to EMS personnel while responding in transit. A simpler "low-tech" solution would be for EMS personnel to ask for an EIF or similar document upon arrival at the home of the patient. Sidebar 7-1, page 122, outlines the AAP's recommendations on formulating an emergency care plan for children with special needs.[6]

TABLE 7-1

Emergency Information Form
for Children with Special Needs

Emergency Information Form for Children With Special Needs

Last name:

	American College of Emergency Physicians®	American Academy of Pediatrics		Date form completed	Revised	Initials
				By Whom	Revised	Initials

Name: | Birth date: | Nickname:

Home Address: | Home/Work Phone:

Parent/Guardian: | Emergency Contact Names & Relationship:

Signature/Consent*:

Primary Language: | Phone Number(s):

Physicians:

Primary care physician: | Emergency Phone:
| Fax:

Current Specialty physician:
Specialty: | Emergency Phone:
| Fax:

Current Specialty physician:
Specialty: | Emergency Phone:
| Fax:

Anticipated Primary ED: | Pharmacy:

Anticipated Tertiary Care Center:

Diagnoses/Past Procedures/Physical Exam:

1. | Baseline physical findings:

2.

3. | Baseline vital signs:

4.

Synopsis: | Baseline neurological status:

*Consent for release of this form to health care providers

(Continued on next page)

Source: American Academy of Pediatrics Committee on Pediatric Emergency Medicine: Emergency Preparedness for Children With Special Health Care Needs. *Pediatrics* 104(4):53, 1999. Reprinted with permission.

TABLE 7-1

Emergency Information Form
for Children with Special Needs (continued)

Last name:

Diagnoses/Past Procedures/Physical Exam continued:

Medications:

1.

2.

3.

4.

5.

6.

Significant baseline ancillary findings (lab, x-ray, ECG):

Prostheses/Appliances/Advanced Technology Devices:

Management Data:

Allergies: Medications/Foods to be avoided   and why:

1.

2.

3.

Procedures to be avoided   and why:

1.

2.

3.

Immunizations

Dates				
DPT				
OPV				
MMR				
HIB				

Dates				
Hep B				
Varicella				
TB status				
Other				

Antibiotic prophylaxis: Indication: Medication and dose:

Common Presenting Problems/Findings With Specific Suggested Managements

Problem	Suggested Diagnostic Studies	Treatment Considerations

Comments on child, family, or other specific medical issues:

Physician/Provider Signature: **Print Name:**

Source: American Academy of Pediatrics Committee on Pediatric Emergency Medicine: Emergency Preparedness for Children With Special Health Care Needs. *Pediatrics* 104(4):53, 1999. Reprinted with permission.

Sidebar 7-1	AAP Recommendations in Formulating an Emergency Care Plan

The American Academy of Pediatrics published the following recommendations for formulating an emergency care plan:

- A brief, comprehensive summary of information important for hospital or prehospital emergency management of a child with special health care needs should be formulated by the child's caregivers, health care professionals, and all subspecialty providers.

- The summary, or emergency medical data set, should be updated regularly and maintained in an accessible and usable format.

- Parents, other caregivers, and health care professionals should be educated to optimize use of the summary. Parents and other caregivers should be encouraged to take the summary with them for all health care encounters.

- Mechanisms to quickly identify children with special health care needs in an emergency should be established and should be available to local EMS and hospital personnel.

- A universally accepted, standardized form should be used for summaries as described in Tables 1 and 2.

- Advanced directives (many states have a standard form) can be attached to or included in this information form.

- Rapid 24/7 access to the summary should be ensured. Copies should be accessible at home, school, during transportation, and in the emergency department in addition to a copy in the records of treating physicians. Linkage to an emergency telephone number such as 911 dispatch or some other method of assuring rapid access is desirable. Especially important is identification of the most appropriate EMS squad to be called in areas without 911 dispatch. Schools and child care facilities should be encouraged to include the emergency summary as part of a child's individual health plan.

- Confidentiality of the form should be carefully maintained. Parental permission to establish the emergency information form and distribute it to appropriate agencies should be obtained and kept on file with the originator of the form or at a central repository.

Adapted from American Academy of Pediatrics Committee on Pediatric Emergency Medicine: Emergency preparedness for children with special health care needs. *Pediatrics* 104(4):53, 1999. A statement of reaffirmation of this statement was published in *Pediatrics* 122(2):450, 2008. Printed with permission.

In addition to communication with the patient's medical home, ED clinicians receiving a child with special health care needs should always inquire about the presence of a health care summary or emergency information form from patients, or their family members, and be aware that many of these children also wear medical jewelry to provide vital information in an emergency. For example, the MedicAlert® Foundation encourages the use of EIFs for children with special health care needs and distributes medical identification bracelets throughout the world. The foundation serves as a repository of information for children who are registered with it and has a 24-hour emergency response center where health care professionals can obtain necessary health care information.[2]

Case Study 7-1 on page 123 illustrates the ways that the AAP/ACEP standardized information form can help ED clinicians individualize the care provided to children with special health care needs.

Supporting Care Coordination

"What do I look for?"

"What do I do?"

"Who do I call?"[7]

Those are the three crucial questions that need to be asked in an emergency. The caregivers' challenge is to give answers that are easily understood and followed. Only key information that guides subsequent actions should be included. Using simple decision trees, action plan formats, and graphics can be effective. Sidebar 7-2 lists the key information that ED clinicians can apply in developing an action plan to treat children with special health care needs.[7] These items can be included in an EIF.

Children with special health care needs typically have multiple health care providers and these should ideally be coordinated via the medical home or primary care

Case Study 7-1

In an Emergency, Children With Special Needs Require Individual Plans

Emergency care can pose a substantial risk for children with special health care needs. "Many of these kids are 1 in 100, 1,000, or 1 million, with medical problems that are unique to them," explained Robert Wiebe, M.D., F.A.A.P., of Dallas. "We had a child with muscular dystrophy who came into our emergency room in acute respiratory distress," recalled Dr. Wiebe, a prior chair of the AAP Committee on Pediatric Emergency Medicine (COPEM). "This is one of the rare occurrences when oxygen can be an enemy rather than a friend" due to the dynamics of the patient's disease, he said. Medical personnel on duty were not familiar with muscular dystrophy, so "they put him on oxygen, which impaired his respiratory drive and he developed respiratory failure and died."

Another prior COPEM member, pediatric cardiologist Lee Pyles, M.D., F.A.A.P., of Minneapolis, remembered when a child from West Virginia who had a corrective surgical procedure for congenital heart disease, was taken to the ED with a rapid heartbeat. "Medical personnel there wanted to treat the boy with verapamil, as they would an adult, but the child's mother was aware that the treatment 'had the potential to make him very ill,'" Dr. Pyles said. "It took the mom a long time to convince the emergency physician to call a pediatric cardiologist." Dr. Pyles is the lead author of a study describing Minnesota's EMSC demonstration project that created a central repository for EIFs using a web-based access system[1] (see www.memscis.org for more information).

To avoid such frightening scenarios, pediatricians and parents should create an emergency plan, and make sure it's available 24 hours a day for every child with chronic physical, developmental, behavioral, or emotional conditions and medical needs beyond those of typically developing children. Guidelines for creating these emergency plans were first developed by the American Academy of Pediatrics and the American College of Emergency Physicians in a joint policy statement published in 1999, "Emergency Preparedness for Children With Special Health Care Needs,"[2] This policy was reaffirmed in 2008 and an update is expected to be published in 2009.

The statement "helps people to know the important points of how to start a program in their community," Dr. Pyles said. "There are so many rare pediatric diseases, and some of the emergency treatments are really very disease-specific. Dr. Wiebe noted the guidelines could also assist ED professionals caring for special needs children with more common chronic health problems such as "sickle cell patients with their unique histories, and asthmatics with their variety of medicines."

Michael Gerardi, M.D., F.A.C.E.P., F.A.A.P., Board member of the American College of Emerging Physicians, was ACEP's consultant to the Academy on the policy statement.[3] "These children have very complicated histories, and without their extensive medical records available, it's very hard (for ED personnel) to get a handle on what's going on," said Dr. Gerardi.

For him, this issue hits close to home. "I have a son with congenital heart disease," Gerardi said, admitting he's wondered for years whether, if he weren't available, the scars on his son's body would be an adequate warning to physicians of the potential for problems during emergency treatment. "We've all taken care of children with scars on their chest and abdomen, or with a bag full of medicine," Dr. Gerardi said, "and (in an emergency) you frequently just can't quite get enough out of the parents."

Drs. Wiebe, Gerardi, and Pyles are all in agreement that while maintaining patient confidentiality is important, this is superseded by the need to access accurate medical information in a timely fashion to optimize the medical care of the child. EIFs should be updated often by primary care providers in a medical home. Specialists and primary care physicians must communicate to optimize the accuracy of these updates.

References

1. Pyles L.A., Hines C., Patock M., et al.: Development of a web-based database to manage American College of Emergency Physicians/American Academy of Pediatrics emergency information forms. *Acad Emerg Med* 12(3):257–261, 2005.

2. American College of Emergency Physicians. Children with special health care needs. Available at: http://www.acep.org/patients.aspx?id=26128 (accessed Nov. 11, 2007).

3. American Academy of Pediatrics Committee on Pediatric Emergency Medicine: Emergency preparedness for children with special health care needs. *Pediatrics* 104(4):53, 1999. A statement or reaffirmation of this statement was published in *Pediatrics* 122(2): 450, 2008 (doi:10.1542/peds.2008–1427).

Adapted from Zanzola L.: In emergency, children with special needs require individual plans. *AAP News,* Oct 1999. Reprinted with permission.

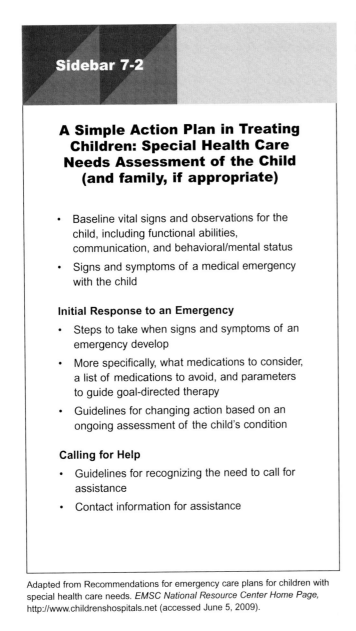

Adapted from Recommendations for emergency care plans for children with special health care needs. *EMSC National Resource Center Home Page,* http://www.childrenshospitals.net (accessed June 5, 2009).

physician. The term "care coordination" is more appropriate than "case management" because parents and families play a significant role in the medical care planning and decision making for children with special health care needs.[8] Care coordination is particularly important in the ED because the ED physician is generally new to the patient's care and may not be fully cognizant of the child's unique health care needs. Optimal emergency care relies on both family members and primary care physicians to communicate information to emergency care personnel.[9,10] Although there remains no standard definition of care coordination in children, a useful foundation for this is provided by the AAP. A 2005 updated policy statement by the AAP Council on Children with Disabilities suggested that care coordination occurs when care plans are implemented by a variety of service providers and programs

in an organized fashion.[8] The statement goes on to present the goals for care coordination as follows[8]:

- Develop an anticipatory/proactive plan for appropriate services for the child and family, integrating the recommendations of multiple professionals and service systems.
- Assist the family in accessing needed services and resources.
- Facilitate communication among multiple professionals.
- Avoid duplication of services and unnecessary costs.
- Optimize the physical and emotional health and well-being of the child.
- Improve the child's and family's quality of life.

Collaborating With the Families of Patients

All aspects of emergency care should be family-centered.[9,10] In some cases, it is the family and not the physician that serves as the primary point of care coordination. The parents of children with special needs are often very well versed on their child's medical condition, special devices, history, and prognosis. In various health care settings, many of these parents have served as volunteer mentors to novice parents whose children are suffering from similar debilitations. Health care professionals need to recognize the parents of children with special needs as equal partners in the emergency care process and encourage them to be part of critical health care decisions.[11]

Families must often balance the intensive needs of their medically fragile child with ongoing daily responsibilities of earning a living, caring for other children, and maintaining a household. Opportunities for time alone and/or time to build personal relationships and social support networks are often severely limited. Studies have shown that up to 70% of mothers and 40% of fathers of severely disabled children experience high levels of distress.[12,13]

Both the costs and enormous time demands associated with the care of their special needs child significantly decrease job security and increase the risk of unemployment and poverty, thereby contributing to greater psychosocial stress and anxiety.[13] This added stress and anxiety may also affect cognitive, behavioral, and social development of disabled or chronically ill children.[14,15]

Depending on the disability and specific condition, children with disabilities are 1.6 to 4 times more likely to be victims of neglect, physical abuse, emotional abuse, or sexual abuse than children without disabilities[16-18] mainly due to caregivers feeling "burnt out," frustrated, and even resentful of their intensive and often overwhelming responsibilities.[17,18] Although truly grasping the perspective of a parent of a child with special needs is impossible without personal experience, simply considering the steps involved in preparing a chronically ill child for a visit to the ED might shed empathetic light on the challenges they face every day. Many parents will bypass the nearest ED to travel to one that they believe can better meet their child's needs.

Managing Devices and Equipment Malfunction in Special Needs Children

Emergency care personnel are often called on to assess the function of medical devices and to perform procedures that are usually done by outpatient specialized care providers.[19] Managing and, if needed, replacing a poorly functioning tracheostomy tube can be a life-saving intervention. Replacing a dislodged or leaking gastrostomy tube, inserting a peritoneal dialysis catheter, repairing a broken central venous access catheter, and assessing the function of a ventriculoperitoneal shunt are examples of skills that are performed by emergency department personnel because these devices will often require immediate attention at times other than office hours. Many of these tasks are not technically difficult; indeed, many can be safely done by trained family members in the home setting. However, for those who are unfamiliar with these devices, particularly in the pediatric population, this may be challenging.

The clinical information and technical skills required to assess, manage, and replace many of these devices are well described in many pediatric emergency care textbooks and review articles.[19-22] A pediatric subspecialist can describe and explain the procedure by phone. What are often lacking are the proper supplies and, of course, ongoing experience, particularly in EDs that care for small numbers of pediatric patients. ED managers should assure that their facility is prepared with the appropriate types and sizes of these devices, reflective of the population of special needs children served, the availability of subspecialty care services at their hospital and local pediatric tertiary care centers. ED staff must also be prepared through ongoing professional education, skills sessions, and the creation of clinical pathways to guide ED care providers what to do and, likewise, what not to do. For children dependent on devices that are known to periodically fail, such as a gastrostomy or tracheostomy tube, it is best to provide parents with replacement devices that they can keep with them. This reduces the likelihood that the correct size or type of a device will be unavailable when it is needed.

Inexpensive devices that are malfunctioning such as a home nebulizer machines are more easily replaced than repaired. Other devices are more complex and will require the expertise of a technician or a physician specialist. For example, managing a home ventilator, an oxygen concentrator, a drug infusion device, analyzing an internal pacemaker, and so on are tasks that are unfamiliar to most emergency care personnel. Every ED should identify in advance the local resources available for technical support and/or replacement of medical equipment.

Developing a Disaster Plan for Children With Special Needs

The origin or type of a disaster, and their frequency, are often geographic-specific. Many communities recognize the types of natural disasters that are most likely to affect them. Some disaster types might be more variable and unexpected but, regardless of the type of disaster, common infrastructure elements are affected. Lack of shelter, water, food, medication, electricity/medical technology, communications, and information technology are common elements that are potentially the consequence of any type of major disaster. Children with special health care needs are especially affected by lack of medication, information technology, and electricity. Preparing for these consequences requires planning and medical assistance.

- Essential chronic medications necessitate a reserve allocation of medication. Medications outdate and insurance companies are usually reluctant to supply a reserve in planning for a rare event. Patients will likely need help to obtain and properly manage a medication reserve.

- Medical management information is often dependent on access to a medical record, which might not be available even electronically if the communication and information infrastructure is compromised. An updated AAP/ACEP EIF printed on water-resistant paper could serve as a valuable source of information in such circumstances.

- For technology-dependent children, loss of electrical power threatens their technology device assistance. Acute high priority life-support devices such as a ventilator or oxygen concentrator must have a built-in battery back-up, which is temporary and must soon be replaced by an alternate longer term source of power that must also power lower priority devices such as a home nebulizer machine or feeding pump. Training parents to provide alternate electrical power by using an automobile inverter or a home generator can be a valuable method of extending the provision of electrical power during a power failure. Depending on a hospital for electrical power is unreliable because the disaster or traffic might impact access and the hospital's limited resources might require it to lock down in order to maintain its ability to care for its patients.

Of the above, electrical power failure is by far the most common disaster impacting medically complex patients. A natural disaster is not necessary for electrical power to fail. A fallen utility pole, a vehicle collision into a power transmission junction, generator malfunction, bad weather, power surges, brown-outs, rotating black-outs, and overgrown trees can all disrupt electrical power. Most physicians are not trained to teach patients how to operate alternate electrical power sources. Organized medicine should recognize that this is the most common threat to technology-dependent patients and develop a standardized training module to address this. Chapter 8 will provide a broader perspective on the consideration of pediatric patient care needs in disaster planning.

Resources for Emergency Care Providers

Medical organizations such as the American Academy of Pediatrics, the American College of Emergency Physicians, the Emergency Nurses Association, and the American Heart Association, and federal programs such as Emergency Medical Services for Children and the Institute of Medicine have assembled an impressive and useful collection of resources that facilitate the collective works of knowledge experts on issues relating to the emergency care of children with special health care needs.

- **SCOPE:** Special Children's Outreach and Prehospital Education is an instructional program developed by EMSC targeted for prehospital emergency care providers. It provides basic information on various chronic medical conditions, technology, and equipment-dependent children and is designed to augment the knowledge and comfort level of prehospital providers when treating and transporting children with special health care needs.[23]

- **PEPP:** Pediatric Education for Prehospital Providers is an instructional program and book developed by the American Academy of Pediatrics. It offers a wide-ranging series of educational resources in pediatric prehospital care, including information on children with special health care needs. This is an ongoing, continuously improving, and developing program maintained by the American Academy of Pediatrics.[24,25]

- **ENPC:** Emergency Nursing Pediatric Course is a 16-hour course developed by the Emergency Nurses Association designed to provide core-level pediatric knowledge and psychomotor skills needed to care for pediatric patients in the emergency setting. The course presents a systematic assessment model, integrates the associated anatomy, physiology, and pathophysiology, and identifies appropriate interventions. Triage categorization and prevention strategies are included in the course content. ENPC is taught using a variety of formats, including lectures, videotapes, and includes skill stations that encourage participants to integrate their psychomotor abilities into a patient situation in a risk-free setting.[26]

- **APLS:** Advanced Pediatric Life Support is an instructional program and textbook developed jointly by the American Academy of Pediatrics and the American College of Emergency Physicians. Previously known as the "pediatric emergency medicine course," its current focus is to be a comprehensive, yet compact informational resource covering the major areas of pediatric emergency care including children with special health care needs. The target audience for APLS are physicians, but the information within the components of the course are useful for emergency nurses and prehospital providers as well.[27,28]

- **PALS:** Pediatric Advanced Life Support is a textbook and a course developed and supported jointly by the American Academy of Pediatrics and the American Heart Association. The traditional focus for PALS has been to provide evidence-based recommendations for pediatric resuscitation. This course is widely attended by physicians, nurses, and prehospital providers.[29]

- **Emergency Care for Children:** Growing Pains (Future of Emergency Care) is a detailed report published in 2006 by the Institute of Medicine on the status of pediatric emergency care in the United States. This report is one component of a three-part report, "Future of the Emergency Care in the U.S. Health Care System."[30] The other two components address the status of hospital-based emergency care[31] and prehospital emergency medical services[32] in the United States.

It should also be noted that although this chapter specifically relates to treating children with special health care needs in the ED, there are emergency conditions in which the patient may be unable to reach an ED. This is most evident during a community or environmental disaster[33] during which it will be difficult to get to the ED, or the ED will be overwhelmed. Some of the above resources address disaster planning and a new focus of the updated AAP/ACEP EIF and joint policy statement addresses this as well. The EMSC National Resource Center has also published a resource to address this.[34]

References

1. McPherson M., Arango P., Fox H., et al.: A new definition of children with special health care needs. *Pediatrics* 102:137–140, 1998.

2. American College of Emergency Physicians: Children with special health care needs. Available at: http://www.acep.org/ patients.aspx?id=26128 (accessed Nov. 11, 2007).

3. American Academy of Pediatrics Committee on Pediatric Emergency Medicine: Emergency preparedness for children with special health care needs. *Pediatrics* 104(4):53, 1999. A statement or reaffirmation of this statement was published in *Pediatrics* 122(2):450, 2008 (doi:10.1542/peds.2008-1427).

4. Pyles L.A., Hines C., Patock M., et al.: Development of a web-based database to manage American College of Emergency Physicians/American Academy of Pediatrics emergency information forms. *Acad Emerg Med* 12(3):257–261, 2005.

5. Emergency Medical Services for Children, National Task Force on Children with Special Health Care Needs: EMS for children: Recommendations for coordinating care for children with special health care needs. *Ann Emerg Med* 30:274–280, 1997.

6. National Center for Education in Maternal and Child Health: Emergency Medical Services for Children: Abstracts of Active Projects FY 1994. Arlington, VA: National Center for Education in Maternal and Child Health, 1994.

7. EMSC National Resource Center. Recommendations for emergency care plans for children with special health care needs. Available at: http://www.childrenshospitals.net/AM/ Template.cfm?Section=Homepage&TEMPLATE=/CM/Content Display.cfm&CONTENTID=27834 (accessed Nov. 15, 2007).

8. Lipkin P.H., Alexander J., Cartwright J.D., American Academy of Pediatrics Council on Children with Disabilities: Care coordination in the medical home: Integrating health and related systems of care for children with special health care needs. *Pediatrics* 116(5):1238–1244, 2005.

9. American Academy of Pediatrics Committee on Pediatric Emergency Medicine, American College of Emergency Physicians Pediatric Emergency Medicine Committee: Patient- and family-centered care and the role of the emergency physician providing care to a child in the emergency department. *Pediatrics* 118(5): 2242–2244, 2006.

10. O'Malley P.J., Brown K., Krug S.E., American Academy of Pediatrics Committee on Pediatric Emergency Medicine: Patient- and family-centered care of children in the emergency department. *Pediatrics* 122(2): e511–521, 2008.

11. Wharton R.H., Levine K.R., Buka S., Emanuel L.: Advance care planning for children with special health care needs: A survey of parental attitudes. *Pediatrics* 97(5):682–687, 1996.

12. McNally S., Ben-Shlomo Y., Newman S.: The effects of respite care on informal carers' well-being: a systematic review. *DisabilRehabilitation* 21(1):1–14, 1999.

13. Sloper P., Turner S.: Risk and resistance factors in the adaption of parents of children with severe physical disability. *J Child Psychol Psychat* 34(2):167–188, 1993.

14. Neufeld S.M., Query B., Drummond J.E.: Respite care users who have children with chronic conditions: Are they getting a break? *J Pediatr Nurs* 16(4):234–244, 2001.

15. Gupta A., Nidhi S.: Psychosocial support for families of children with autism. *Asia Pacific Disabil Rehabil J* 16(2):62–83, 2005.

16. Hazell P.L., Tarren-Sweeney M., Vimpani G.V., et al.: Children with disruptive behaviors clinical and community service needs. *J Pediatric Child Health* 38:32–40, April 2001.

17. Sullivan P.M., Knutson J.F.: Maltreatment and disabilities: A Population-based epidemiological study. *Child Abuse Neglect* 24(10):1257–1273, 2000.

18. American Academy of Pediatrics, Committee on Child Abuse and Neglect, Committee on Children with Disabilities: Assessment of maltreatment of children with disabilities. *Pediatrics* 108(2):508–512, 2001.

19. Theo D.L.: Tricks of the trade: assessment of high-tech gear in special needs children. *Clan Pediatric Emerge Med* 3:62–75, 2002.

20. Fleisher G.R., Ludwig S., Heretic F., et al. (eds.): *Textbook of Pediatric Emergency Medicine,* 5th ed. Philadelphia, PA: Lippincott, Williams & Wilkins, 2005.

21. King C., Henretig F., King B., Loiselle J., Ruddy R. (eds.). *Textbook of Pediatric Emergency Procedures,* 2nd ed. Philadelphia, PA: Lippincott, Williams & Wilkins, 2005.

22. Baren J., Rothrock S., Brennan J., Brown L.: *Pediatric Emergency Medicine.* Philadelphia, PA: W.B. Saunders, 2007.

23. Adirim T., Smith E.B. *Special Children's Outreach and Prehospital Education (SCOPE).* Sudbury, MA: Jones and Bartlett Publishers, Inc., 2006. ISBN-13: 9780763724689, ISBN-10: 0763724688.

24. American Academy of Pediatrics: Pediatric Education for Prehospital Professionals (PEPP). Available at: http://www.peppsite.com/about.cfm (accessed Nov. 2, 2008).

25. Brownstein D. (ed.): *Pediatric Education for Prehospital Professionals,* 2nd ed., Elk Grove Village, IL: American Academy of Pediatrics, 2005.

26. Emergency Nurses Association: Emergency Nursing Pediatric Course. Available at: http://www.ena.org/catn_enpc_tncc/enpc/.

27. American Academy of Pediatrics, American College of Emergency Physicians: APLS: The Pediatric Emergency Medicine Resource, 4th ed. Available at: http://www.aplsonline.com/ (accessed Nov. 2, 2008).

28. Fuchs S., Gausche-Hill M., Yamamoto L. (eds.): American Academy of Pediatrics and American College of Emergency Physicians: *APLS: The Pediatric Emergency Medicine Resource,* 4th ed. Sudbury, MA: Jones and Bartlett Publishers, Inc., 2007. ISBN-13: 978-0-7637-4414-4, ISBN-10: 0-7637-4414-X.

29. Ralston M., Hazinski M.F., Zaritsky A.L., et al. (eds.): American Heart Association and American Academy of Pediatrics: PALS Course Guide and PALS Provider Manual: Provider Manual (Paperback). Dallas, TX: American Heart Association, 2007. ISBN-10: 0874935288, ISBN-13: 9780874935288.

30. Institute of Medicine Committee on the Future of Emergency Care in the United States Health System: Emergency Care for Children: Growing Pains. Washington, D.C.: National Academies Press, 2007. ISBN-10: 0309101719, ISBN-13: 978-0309101714.

31. Institute of Medicine Committee on the Future of Emergency Care in the United States Health System: Hospital-Based Emergency Care—At the Breaking Point. Washington, D.C.: National Academy Press, 2006.

32. Institute of Medicine Committee on the Future of Emergency Care in the United States Health System: Emergency Medical Services—At The Crossroads. Washington, D.C.: National Academy Press, 2006.

33. Dolan M.A., Krug S.E.: Pediatric disaster preparedness in the wake of Katrina: lessons to be learned. *Clin Pediatr Emerg Med* 7(1):59–66, 2006.

34. U.S. Department of Health and Human Services. Health Resources and Services Administration: Disaster Preparedness Planning for Children and Youth with Special Health Care Needs. Available at: http://bolivia.hrsa.gov/emsc/Downloads/DisasterPrepCSHCN/DisasterPreparednessforCSHCN.htm (accessed Nov. 2, 2008).

CHAPTER 8

Including Pediatric Care Needs in Disaster Management

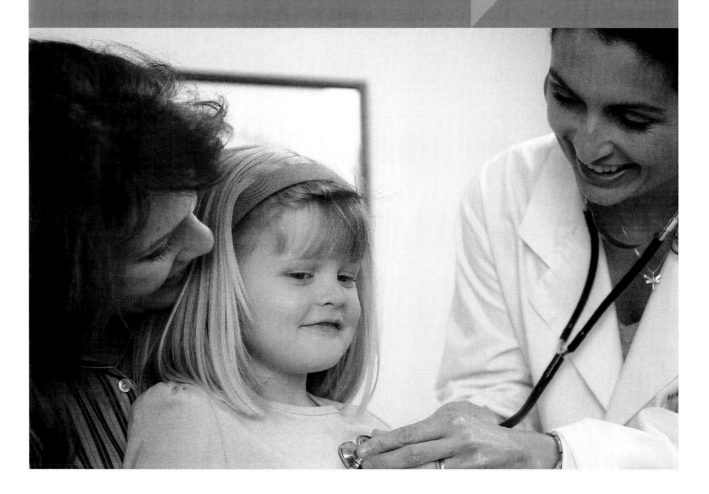

Authored by Francine Westergaard, R.N., M.S.N.,
M.B.A., consultant, Joint Commission Resources and Joint
Commission International; and Mary Lacher, M.D.,
F.A.A.P., intermittent consultant, Joint Commission Resources
and attending physician, Dayton Children's Hospital; and
Steven E. Krug, M.D., F.A.A.P., Head of the Division of
Emergency Medicine, Children's Memorial Hospital, Chicago

Hospitals must be fully prepared to meet the needs of the community they serve when a disaster strikes. Disaster planning must encompass all potential hazards, both naturally occurring (e.g., tornado, hurricane, flood, earthquake, pandemic flu) and manmade, including acts of terrorism. Mass casualty events, whether natural or manmade, will likely involve children. Unfortunately, certain mass casualty events, whether by accident or by design, may primarily target children.

During a disaster, children will present to hospitals based on their location relative to the event, and some of these hospitals may have limited pediatric capabilities. All hospitals must be prepared to accurately triage pediatric victims, implement decontamination when indicated, and provide initial stabilization and emergency treatment for children of all ages.[1–3] The scope or type of disaster may also require hospitals to provide ongoing medical care for disaster victims, including children, for several days until transfer and transportation can be arranged. This requires hospitals to consider a surge capacity and capability plan that includes pediatric care needs. This chapter will provide an overview of pediatric care needs that should be considered in hospital disaster planning.

Understanding the Unique Differences in the Pediatric Patient

Children possess distinctive needs in regards to their unique anatomic, physiologic, developmental, and psychological characteristics. There are also social and environmental needs that should be considered in preparing to care for children and their families during and after a mass casualty event. These differences make children among the most vulnerable populations in the event of a disaster.[1–5] Children, especially those under five, have an increased mortality rate in disasters compared to adults.[6]

Anatomic and Physiologic Differences

Specific anatomic and physiologic differences need to be taken into consideration when caring for the pediatric disaster victim.[3,7] Children are more likely to sustain greater damage from inhalation in a fire or from an aerosolized biological or chemical agent.[8,9] Children take more breaths per minute compared to adults and their "breathing zone" is closer to the ground where toxins that are heavier than air tend to gather, thereby giving them a higher toxic load. Due to a smaller airway diameter, mild degrees of airway swelling from an inhalation insult, or from an upper airway infection, can cause partial or complete airway obstruction. Hospitals must be prepared to manage this acute life-threatening problem with professionals competent to provide safe pediatric care and have adequate supplies of pediatric-sized airway equipment and the medications used to treat airway concerns in the pediatric patient.[1]

Children also have a proportionately larger body surface area and thinner skin, which makes them more prone to dermal absorption of chemicals or radiation and, therefore, may experience greater toxic effects from these agents.[8–14] Timely decontamination at the scene, or immediately

upon arrival to the hospital, is therefore more crucial for children.[2,15] As will be discussed later in this chapter, the decontamination of children requires special considerations. The presence of a relatively large surface area to body mass ratio creates a greater risk for hypothermia in children.[2,3] Hypothermia can be an unfortunate byproduct of decontamination, or can result from prolonged exposure in an emergency department (ED) examination room.

The pediatric patient is also more prone to the development of shock. Although they can compensate for hypovolemia for longer periods of time than adults, children have a smaller blood volume and less fluid reserves compared to adult patients.[16,17] Children therefore have a greater risk for shock resulting from traumatic blood loss or from dehydration secondary to vomiting and diarrhea caused by an infectious agent or toxin. Compared to adults, children are more likely to sustain a serious injury and concomitant blood loss from blast injuries, as their smaller size results in the force of the blast being distributed over a smaller surface, hence a greater net force.[18] This, combined with the proximity of organs in children, results in more multi-organ involvement. Finally, due to their body size proportions, children are also much more likely to sustain head trauma from blasts or other blunt injury mechanisms. This is an important consideration as the presence and severity of head injury is commonly the primary determinant of functional outcome for injured children and must be considered during the triage process.[19,20]

Emergency and disaster care providers who are not experienced with treating children may miss the early signs of shock in the pediatric patient. These signs include an increase in the heart and respiratory rate, a decrease in perfusion, and weakening peripheral pulses.[16,17] The decrease in blood pressure that is seen earlier on in the evolution of shock in adults is typically a very late sign of shock in the pediatric patient. For the pediatric patient, normal baseline vital signs cover a wide range based on the patient's age. Because changes in vital signs are one of the earliest signs in shock, these clues will be missed if health care providers are not knowledgeable of age-based norms for vital signs. Ready access to pediatric vital sign resources (see Table 6-1, on page 98) will be invaluable to health care providers in their assessment and treatment of the pediatric patient.

Developmental and Psychological Differences

Developmental issues can place children at a greater risk during a disaster event.[3,6,7] Young children lack the cognitive abilities and self-preservation skills to know how to respond or react in a dangerous situation. Developmentally, children may also lack the necessary motor skills to escape from a dangerous environment. It may also be difficult for children to understand or follow the directions of a "stranger" who is trying to help them. Their imagination and lack of comprehension of the events around them may impede the efforts of those who are trying to assist and help them. For example, imagine how a pre-school-aged child would perceive emergency responders in biohazard gear giving them instructions.

Children are at significant risk for the development of acute and post-traumatic stress responses following disasters.[3,6,21-25] This has been observed in the aftermath of natural disasters and acts of terror. Surveys of grade-school students conducted six months after major hurricanes have noted a surprisingly high prevalence of post-traumatic stress disorders, with reports indicating that more than 90% of children demonstrated at least mild symptoms, 50% to 70% experienced moderate symptoms, and 30% to 40% demonstrated severe symptoms. The incidence and severity of these concerns may likely be greater after an act of terror. Although symptoms relating to acute and post-traumatic stress disorders may not be a component of the acute presentation of victims immediately after a disaster, families should be made aware of this fairly common complication, and staff should be trained to recognize symptoms in patients at risk, particularly in caring for children and families in the aftermath of a disaster. As less than 30% of children in New York City who suffered severe or very severe post-traumatic stress reactions following 9/11 received counseling services, the ED presentation of children suffering from untreated psychological disorders following a disaster should be anticipated.[26] Staff should be prepared to educate families regarding this important issue and prepare them for the likelihood of its occurrence. Recent survey data indicates that there is a need for improved awareness and education for emergency care professionals and even among pediatric emergency care specialists.[27]

The pediatric patient is also at risk for "nosocomial trauma." This type of trauma may occur after the disaster and may be an unintended consequence of the disaster response and treatment. Exposure to increased psychological stress, physical injury, separation from family and familiar surroundings, and being placed in a hectic, frightening environment may contribute to this type of trauma. As an example, if the reactions of those caring for the child (and many others) are stressed and the care setting is chaotic,

this will add to the trauma already inflicted on the child from the original event. Besides the emergency care or the "physical first aid" that the child may require, there will likely be a need for "psychological first aid."[21] For those not accustomed to working with children, recognizing this need and having a plan or process to provide support may be a challenging task. Yet, in order to have the pediatric patient's and family members' cooperation to deal with their medical needs, one must also address their emotional needs as well.

During a disaster, children may present to a health care facility unaccompanied by an adult or family member. In these circumstances, the psychological stress is greatly increased as most children are very dependent on support provided by parents and family when they are ill or injured. A primary goal in caring for unaccompanied children should be to reunite them with family members as quickly as possible. Providing reassurance to the unaccompanied child that such efforts are ongoing may prove to be comforting. An unaccompanied child can easily become frightened by the activities that occur during emergency care, and these stressors may be greater still with the urgency imposed by a disaster event. Interactions with multiple public safety personnel and disaster care providers, conducting invasive assessments and potentially painful procedures, can be overwhelming for children of all ages. Disaster response leadership should evaluate the organization's plan with a goal to identify a role for an adult staff member to remain with unaccompanied children to provide comfort and reassurance.

Parents that accompany their child will need insight and assistance from emergency care providers in how best to recognize and respond to psychological trauma and how to keep secondary trauma (e.g., vivid media accounts of the disaster event) to a minimum. If the parents are also suffering from psychological trauma, or are simply stressed and upset, these emotions will be picked up by the child. Providing timely information to the parents about the care needs and condition of their ill or injured child can go a long way in reducing their fear and stress level and may help in directing them to assist in the acute care of their child.

Children are also at a higher risk than adults for the evolution of hysteria. This can be especially problematic when caring for a group of children. In this situation, it is crucial for the pediatric patient to immediately experience calm adults who know how to effectively communicate what is happening to them. The adults need to be caring, reassuring, and able to explain the situation to the child and the care process that the child will experience.

Addressing the Needs of Unaccompanied Children and Families

Hurricane Katrina highlighted the unique social service needs of children during evacuation and sheltering. A chaotic evacuation plan, combined with the enormous impact of the storm, resulted in hundreds of children being displaced from their homes and families.[6,28] The Katrina experience emphasizes the importance of planning for the identification and appropriate supervision of unaccompanied children and similarly for coordinated efforts aimed toward timely reunification with family.[21,22,29] Photographs of unaccompanied pediatric patients (including those who have died) can be extremely helpful in identifying children and reuniting them with their families.[29,30] This is especially true for pre-verbal children. Hospital disaster plans should contain a process for the creation of temporary identifiers for unaccompanied children and the timely communication of this information to appropriate agencies (e.g., law enforcement, social services, National Center for Missing and Exploited Children). These processes should define the necessary components for temporary identification (key physical descriptors, where the child was located/found), and ideally should incorporate a digital image that can be used to track the child throughout the process of care.[30]

For children that have been medically cleared, the disaster plan must consider how unaccompanied children will be managed until they have been reunited with family or released to local authorities for evacuation or sheltering.[31] As has been implemented during recent disaster events by the Save the Children Federation, a "pediatric safe area" providing appropriate adult supervision, safety, and security should be established in the organization where children (and intact families) can be kept safely and away from the chaos of acute treatment areas.[32] Temporary treatment and sheltering facilities must anticipate the needs of children of all ages, addressing nutrition (i.e., formula), clothing, (appropriate sizes), sanitation (i.e., diapers), and even safe sleeping (i.e., cribs) accommodations. Ideally, these areas can be staffed by personnel (e.g., child life, social service, chaplains, volunteers) who can assist patients and families in addressing psychosocial needs.

An area away from the media should be set up for family members of disaster victims, where staff can go to have private conversations with family to keep them informed of events. Such "family areas" were utilized by hospitals during Hurricane Katrina. Parents found support from family members of other children in the same situation and received aid from other families, including transportation

assistance, when multiple families had children transferred to different facilities.[33] Hospitals should consider a family information and support center as a component of their disaster planning.[34]

For unaccompanied children that require admission to the hospital, disaster plans should also consider the use of "sitters" as it is likely that available clinical staff will not have the time to provide adequate supervision, particularly for younger children. This may be especially important if the surge capacity plan requires the use of adult patient designed facilities for pediatric care and, as an example, the use of an adult patient bed rather than a crib for an infant or toddler. Therefore, disaster surge response considerations for the care of children in adult facilities should encompass an assessment of the environment and the inherent safety risks.[34]

Children and adults with special health care needs will also be affected by disasters, and hospital disaster plans must consider the needs of this at-risk population.[35] The simple loss of power may serve as a disaster-like event for patients and their families that rely on utilities to support medical technology.[36,37] Hospitals and other facilities with emergency power capabilities will be viewed as a "life line" by technology dependent patients. Hospitals should anticipate this and plan for the maintenance of patients presenting to their ED who need access to electricity, or to equipment, medications, and supplies that were left at home or were damaged or lost due to the disaster. Hospitals may need to provide medical supplies (oxygen tanks, nebulizer machines, ventilator supplies, medications, etc.) to such displaced patients and families.

Planning for Children in a Mass Casualty Event

No matter what the cause, there is a high probability that children will be involved in a disaster event. Health care facilities must therefore be prepared to manage pediatric patients as part of their planning. Preparedness for children of all ages is likely to be facilitated through the involvement of pediatricians in all aspects of planning.[1] Disaster plans should include a needs assessment that reflects the community a hospital serves and an analysis of hazard vulnerability.[2,38] Planning should consider the potential for the direct impact of the event on the hospital facility and the need and means for patient evacuation. Health facility plans also must be coordinated within the emergency management plan for the community or region. These disaster plans should be evaluated and refined based on rigorous testing and drills. Lastly, emergency management performance measures are necessary to evaluate the status of an organization's disaster readiness (e.g. resources, surge capacity), as well as efforts to improve readiness after a drill or actual event. These measures must also address the unique care needs of children.

Pediatric disaster planning begins in the community and pre-hospital environment and must be maintained through the continuum of care. Planning for pediatric victims begins with the appropriate preparation of local first responders and by teams, such as DMATs (Disaster Medical Assistance Teams), that are mobilized by the National Disaster Medical System.[39] Since 9/11 there has been significant attention directed toward pre-hospital preparedness, but gaps still remain in pediatric emergency management and disaster readiness.[40] In a survey of disaster readiness of EMS programs, Shirm and colleagues found that only 13% of pre-hospital agencies reported an adequate, pediatric-specific, mass-casualty plan.[41] Many of the organizations surveyed did not have a plan for caring for children with special health care needs. In addition, less than 20% of those responding indicated their planned use of a pediatric triage tool. Findings such as these indicate obvious gaps in readiness for children and serve as a reminder of the 2006 IOM report, which noted that there was still much work to be done to improve our preparation for pediatric victims of mass-casualty events.[40]

Hospital plans should consider nearby schools and daycare centers as part of their hazard vulnerability assessment.[2,38] Because children spend a large majority of their time at school or in day care centers, certain events could result in many children requiring the services of the hospital. Although many school systems now report that they have developed a disaster plan, gaps still remain in school readiness for day-to-day emergencies and mass-casualty events. In a survey conducted in 2004, Graham and colleagues found that nearly one-third of schools had not conducted a disaster drill and one-fifth had made no provisions for special needs children.[42] Almost half of the responding schools had not met with local EMS agencies to discuss their plan. Surveys of school readiness for day-to-day emergencies involving children indicate related opportunities to improve school plans.[43]

Hospitals should partner with local schools, EMS, and pediatric care providers in the community to assist schools to improve their emergency and disaster readiness. This outreach may also prove to be useful for hospital resource planners, as a well-developed and integrated plan at local

schools may serve to reduce unneeded use of the hospital's limited acute care resources by patients who may not need those services. Hospitals may find it possible to partner with schools, particularly those that are nearby, for use of the school's facilities as a temporary shelter for patients who have been screened and need no additional care. School staff may be ideally suited to work with frightened children during a time of great stress, and schools may prove to be an ideal safe location to house children and families and possibly groups of unaccompanied children.

Hospital planners should also partner with pediatric care providers in the community. Primary care pediatricians and pediatric surgical and medical specialists are ideally suited to assist hospitals in developing emergency response plans and disaster surge capacity and capability plans that will address the needs of children. Pediatricians should be engaged in all aspects of hospital disaster planning and, likewise, in local community and state disaster planning.[1,4-6,19] Hospitals also have a shared interest in partnering with community-based care providers in an effort to maintain access to the medical home in the immediate aftermath of a disaster, as this may help to limit unneeded use of hospital acute care (e.g., ED) resources. As was the case following Hurricane Katrina, there may also be a role for hospitals to provide assistance to local emergency planners in caring for large numbers of disaster victims who have been evacuated for sheltering.[44,45]

The hospital's plan should define roles and responsibilities for staff members and outline operational policies to be activated during a disaster. Emergency department personnel and other hospital staff providing care to pediatric disaster victims and their families cannot carry out these roles without adequate, ongoing training. Readiness for pediatric mass-casualty events can be achieved only if it is built on a foundation of preparedness for day-to-day emergency care.[1,38,46] Hospital EDs should strive to meet published guidelines for pediatric emergency readiness as advocated by the Emergency Medical Services for Children program and several professional organizations, including the American Academy of Pediatrics, the American College of Emergency Physicians and the Emergency Nurses Association.[1,40,47] Disaster care requires the acquisition of knowledge and the development of skills to address medical needs resulting from all potential hazards. Disaster education and training similarly must also encompass the emotional, social, and psychological needs of children and their families. These are skills that an organization must recognize as essential and staff should be provided with the opportunities to pursue this education and training.

Staff must also be provided an opportunity to "exercise" and further improve their skills through drills.

There is also a need to educate and train those who will assume leadership positions during a mass-casualty event. Representatives from all aspects of the hospital must be involved in the organization's disaster planning so they can appreciate the special needs of children during a disaster. These individuals must understand their roles and responsibilities during crisis management. A key responsibility of leadership is coordinating disaster drills as a means to challenge and improve the system. Drills should always include pediatric victims, and organizations should engage in one pediatric mass-casualty drill that significantly exceeds the normal number of children typically handled by the hospital at least once every two years.[1,2,40] In assessing pediatric components of the organization's plan, leadership should consider these recommendations from a 2007 National Consensus Conference on pediatric preparedness for disasters and terrorism:[48]

1. Engage in a pediatric-specific disaster risk assessment with the community, including school districts, the Office of Emergency Services, EMS, the police department, private practitioners, child welfare organizations, child care establishments, public health organizations, and mental health facilities.

2. Develop informational resources and training for pediatric-specific responses to biological, chemical, and radiological terrorism.

3. Ensure that all hospital emergency operations and preparedness policies include pediatric care and treatment guidelines and account for the unique aspects and needs of children.

4. Ensure that all agents and equipment that are stocked for disaster and terrorism preparedness are either specifically for pediatric use or can be appropriately substituted for pediatric use.

The Emergency Medical Services for Children strategic plan for 2008–2010 encourages the following disaster planning activities:[47]

1. Review and disseminate guidelines on how to appropriately respond to children and families before, during, and after a disaster at the national, state, and local level.

2. Encourage incorporation of pediatric disaster preparation into initial education, continuing education, and credentialing of emergency medical care providers.

3. Increase the level of pediatric expertise on disaster medical assistance teams and other organized disaster response teams.

4. Review and disseminate disaster plan strategies that address pediatric surge capacity before, during, and after a disaster for both injured and non-injured children at the national, state, and local levels.

Communication

As was clearly demonstrated during Hurricane Katrina, many of the problems encountered in the response to a disaster are embedded in failed communication.[6] Without accurate and reliable communication among the many government agencies, public safety, and disaster response entities and a host of private organizations (including hospitals and other health care organizations) from the very onset of a disaster, chaos will most certainly result and the needs of victims may not be optimally met. Barrier-free and effective communication among these many involved parties during a disaster requires thoughtful advanced planning that defines roles, responsibilities, and expected routes of communication. Advanced planning should consider how the hospital organization will communicate externally with public safety agencies and key disaster responders and within the organization to hospital staff. Disaster planning and external communication should consider local schools and daycare centers, as settings with large numbers of children pose unique disaster readiness needs.

Communication with First Responders

Clear and consistent communication between pre-hospital care providers and the hospital is a must during day-to-day emergency care. This same communication becomes even more crucial when preparing to care for multiple victims, regardless of whether the mass-casualty event is small or large in scale. Effective communication from first responders at the disaster scene with the hospital supports optimal preparation and allocation of resources for arriving victims. Information regarding the number, acuity, and types of patients anticipated provides an opportunity to ensure that appropriate staff and supplies are available to care for patients once they arrive at the hospital.

First responders must have the tools, and ideally some relative experience, that will support accurate acuity assessment of children in the field. Tools such as the Pediatric Assessment Triangle, the Pediatric Triage Tape, and JumpSTART provide prehospital health care professionals with an organized approach to pediatric patient assessment and a triage system that addresses the unique characteristics of children.[49] The use of pediatric-specific triage tools will help to reduce both over- and under-triage of children. As acute care resources are frequently overmatched in a disaster, accurate triage is vital. The utility of pediatric triage tools at the hospital will be discussed later in this chapter.

Communication Within the Hospital

The need for excellent communication within the hospital during an influx of critical patients cannot be overemphasized. As the entrance point during a mass-casualty event, the ED must be in constant contact with first responders to maintain optimal preparation for an influx of pediatric patients. Incident command and hospital leadership must keep the ED updated regarding issues of surge capacity, including the availability of necessary staff, supplies, and space to expand. This may include expanding into ambulatory care exam rooms, recovery areas, or non-clinical space. Equally important, the ED must also keep the hospital command center informed of clinical concerns and resource needs during the event.

It is important for the ED to have a designated individual responsible for coordination of staff and resources within the department during a mass-casualty event. It will be important for this individual to be aware of the constant changes that are occurring within the ED during the rapid influx of patients. This individual will facilitate the ongoing care provided by the health care facility linking pediatric patients with staff who have the appropriate skills and expertise to care for them. There should be a mechanism in place that identifies this person to all staff entering and communicating with the ED.

Communication with Disaster Victims and Families

Children presenting to the ED during a mass-casualty event may not have the cognitive or developmental ability to communicate with those who are caring for them. It will be the staff's responsibility to provide comfort and reassurance while simultaneously providing care and treatment to those that are critically ill. Many health care organizations have plans delegating non-licensed individuals to provide comfort care to children who are stable but in need of minimal assistance. It is likely that some disaster victims will not speak English. Part of the organization's preparations should include methods to communicate with non-English speaking patients and families. Planning should anticipate failed access to resources used in daily operations, such as

translator phone lines, due to the disaster. The hospital's plan should maintain an updated listing of staff who are bi- or multilingual. This information should be readily available to staff in the ED and other departments that will provide care to mass-casualty event victims. The creation of a family information and support center may help to improve the quality and consistency of communication with family members and may also reduce some of the related burden upon acute care providers.[34]

Patient Triage

After a mass-casualty event has occurred, patient triage will occur both at the scene and once again at the hospital.[10,50] There is perhaps no more difficult and no more important setting for triage than during a mass-casualty event. The area or population affected typically may exceed the capacity of local patient care resources, stressing available health care facilities beyond their capabilities. Triage is essential as it prioritizes the allocation of precious resources to those who need them the most and only to those who are likely to survive.[47] For every unsalvageable patient who receives prioritized emergency and critical care, it is estimated that the needs of two to four critical patients (who were salvageable) will go unmet. So, contrary to standard pre-hospital and emergency department triage practices, the most critically ill patients may be bypassed for those who are deemed to be salvageable. Even for the most seasoned emergency care provider this is a very challenging, emotional task, and particularly when the victim is a child.

Many prehospital care providers and many hospital EDs are becoming familiar with the START (Simple Triage And Rapid Treatment) mass-casualty incident triage program.[51] This program triages victims into one of four categories based on defined clinical criteria. These clinical criteria were derived from adult patient populations. When applied to children, START does not appear to be as accurate, with a tendency to both under- and over-triage pediatric patients. As children possess distinct differences from adults in key clinical variables utilized by START (i.e., vital signs) this should not be surprising. Use of appropriate triage tools can prevent under-triage or over-triage and avoid poor outcomes in the high stakes setting of a mass-casualty event.

When triaging children, it is important for decisions to be based on objective data. Many times, emotions can get in the way of objective triage. A pediatric version of the START program was developed by Dr. Lou Romig, a pediatric emergency medicine specialist and expert in disaster medicine. This pediatric triage program is known as JumpSTART.[52] As demonstrated in Figure 8-1, page 137, JumpSTART considers a number of key differences in children. First, it addresses the reality that otherwise healthy infants and very young children may not follow commands or be able to walk when directed to do so. This particular JumpSTART criterion can result in the over-triage of these children. JumpSTART also encourages an effort to resuscitate apneic children, particularly those with a palpable pulse, calling for a brief trial with ventilation. This recognizes the prevalence of reversible upper airway obstruction and primary respiratory failure in children. Finally, JumpStart adopts pediatric vital sign criteria and assessments of perfusion and mental status that are more appropriate for children.

It is critical for disaster victim triage skills to be learned by field and hospital personnel and then reinforced by repetitive practice. Trauma coordinators from the trauma centers in Wisconsin have worked through the state trauma system to promote ongoing training with disaster triage through the implementation of "Triage Tuesday."[53] On Tuesdays, Wisconsin EMS providers are encouraged to triage all transported patients utilizing START and/or JumpSTART and apply an appropriate color tag to each. Hospitals receiving these patients evaluate the triage tags to:

- Determine if the triage tag color codes used by the EMS providers would have been the same triage decision made by the ED staff

- Determine whether the information provided on the triage tag was helpful to the ED staff

- Determine from the ED staff perspective what enhancements can be made to the triage tagging process to help improve patient care in the field, during transport, and at the hospital.[54]

Decontamination

Decontamination of pediatric patients requires special consideration for their unique physiologic and developmental characteristics.[3,10,55,56] Utilizing a process designed for adult victims may not be safe or effective. Because children possess a relatively immature thermoregulatory system, special care must be taken to avoid hypothermia during decontamination, as this can lead to poor patient outcomes. Water temperature must be adjusted so that it is warm and the water supply used should be high volume but low pressure to avoid injury.[57]

Decontamination efforts for pediatric patients can be further complicated by the limitations imposed by the developmental stage of the patient. Infants and other non-ambulatory children will obviously be unable to proceed in a process

reliant upon ambulatory adult patients. Younger children are also not likely to cooperate during decontamination nor will many be able to engage in effective self-decontamination. Decontamination suits worn by health care providers can be very frightening for children. Health care workers wearing protective equipment may have a difficult time being able to communicate with pediatric victims. Signage explaining the decontamination process with pictures detailing and depicting the decontamination process can be helpful, especially for children who cannot read and for those with language barriers.

Consideration should be given to supporting family decontamination if family members present to the emergency department together. Staff must be prepared to assist parents as some may struggle with expectations that they decontaminate themselves and their child. The organization's plan must also have available trained staff to assist in the decontamination of unaccompanied children.[57] On completion of decontamination, staff may need to provide assistance in drying children as this too will reduce the risk of hypothermia. Staff will also need to have child-size gowns or clothing available for the children to wear after they have participated in the decontamination process.

Acute Care Capability and Surge Capacity

Surge capacity refers to a hospital's ability to manage a sudden, unexpected increase in patient volume that would otherwise severely challenge or exceed its normal capacity. Few American hospitals have the capacity to handle the increased volume of patients likely to result from a large-scale disaster or pandemic, particularly if the patients were predominantly infants or small children.[3] With ED overcrowding a nearly daily concern in most communities, hospitals may likely be unable to handle even a small influx of critically ill or injured pediatric patients.

Surge capacity includes the availability of empty beds and the necessary competent hospital staff, appropriate medications, equipment, and other supplies to care for patients within the first few hours to days after a disaster. In general, hospitals should plan to be self-sufficient for a minimum of 72 hours following a major event. The U.S. Health Resources and Services Administration surge capacity benchmark is for 500 hospital beds per one million people. This benchmark does not differentiate pediatric from adult hospital beds. For most hospitals, surge capacity will be more easily achieved for adult patients than pediatric patients as most hospital facilities

FIGURE 8-1

JumpSTART Pediatric MCI Triage

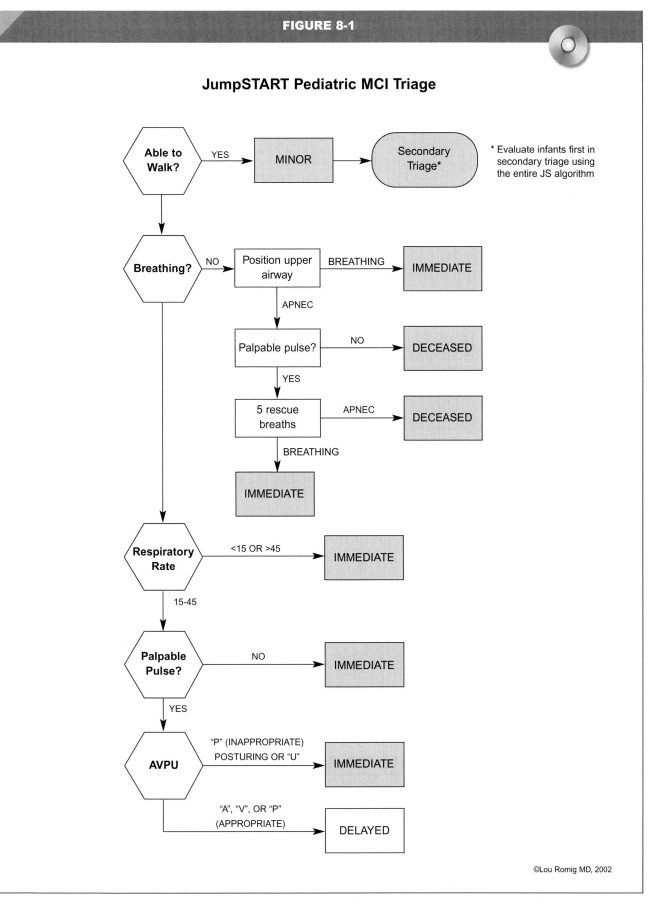

Romig L.E.: Pediatric triage. A system to JumpSTART your triage of young patients at MCIs. *J Emerg Med Serv* 27(7):52-8, 60–63, 2002. Available at http://www.jumpstarttriage.com/. Reprinted with permission.

and hospital-based care providers primarily provide care to adults. Often times, space is not as much of an issue as are readily available pediatric supplies and access to staff with the skills necessary to care for pediatric patients. Although the presence of sufficient amounts of equipment (including pediatric appropriate sizes), medications, and space are clearly important considerations in planning, the rate limiting step in creating surge capacity is the availability of qualified clinical staff.[58]

All available space within the organization, including ambulatory care exam rooms, observation and inpatient beds, even operating rooms, must be considered in surge capacity planning. Pediatric surge capacity plans should be created for all levels of care, including[3]:

- Patient triage and decontamination
- Emergency care and non-emergent acute ambulatory patient care
- Inpatient care—including critical care
- Mental health services

In planning for disasters involving infectious agents, the availability of isolation beds for emergency care and inpatient care will be important, and surge planning might include considerations of the functional isolation of entire patient care units. A vital consideration in planning for mass casualties will be critical care bed space. Many perceive critical care bed availability, and the component technology and specialized staff support (e.g., ventilators and respiratory therapists), to be the greatest deficiency in present-day hospital-based surge capacity. Considering the unique needs of gravely ill children, and the specialized skills required to care for these patients, this weakness would likely be most evident in a pediatric mass-casualty event.

Every hospital's disaster plan should specifically address the issue of pediatric surge capacity and should reflect the unique characteristics of the organization and the presence of pediatric care resources.[58] Typical day-to-day ED clinical practices and referral patterns (hopefully supported by a pediatric specialty transfer agreement) may not be possible during a disaster event. The ability and means to transport patients to a local or regional pediatric tertiary care center may be suspended during a disaster. This will require the hospital to provide care for pediatric patients, including critically ill or injured children, which are ordinarily transferred to another facility. Depending on the type and scope of disaster, hospitals may find that they are obliged to care for these challenging patients for an extended period, and plans must consider this scenario. The local

community or regional disaster plan should include a consideration of the number and type (e.g., critical care, inpatient) of pediatric beds available.

Pediatric Equipment

Hospitalized pediatric patients require appropriate-sized supplies, equipment, and medication formularies that are different than those required by adults. At a minimum, hospitals should endeavor to meet the essential equipment recommendations offered by the American Academy of Pediatrics, American College of Emergency Physicians, and the Emergency Nurses Association for pediatric emergency care (see Sidebar 6-1. Clinical and Professional Competency on page 97).[1] It has been recommended that hospitals maintain a supply of these medications and equipment to meet the needs of the average number of children cared for in a 72-hour period, plus an additional 100 patients.[48] As most hospitals will not stock large amounts of pediatric-sized equipment, arrangements should be made in advance to facilitate timely access to sufficient amounts of these supplies for children in a mass-casualty event. Non-medical supplies necessary for the care of pediatric patients should also be considered,[2,59] including those in Table 8-1 on page 139.

Staff Qualified to Provide Pediatric Care

It is essential for the hospital ED to be staffed by clinicians who are competent in the emergency care of children. During a mass-casualty event, the ED may likely be overwhelmed by the numbers and/or acuity of patients seeking care. An effective disaster plan mobilizes clinical staff from other hospital departments to help meet the needs of disaster victims. The hospital should integrate pediatric patient staffing considerations into its disaster plan and identify staff with pediatric experience and expertise that may be called upon to assist.[60] As there may not be sufficient available staff at the hospital with pediatric care experience, organizations preparing for a pediatric mass casualty will need to expand the size of their pediatric capable workforce through targeted continuing professional education. As recommended by the American Academy of Pediatrics, the American College of Emergency Physicians, and the Emergency Nurses Association, efforts to improve the hospital's readiness for day-to-day pediatric emergency care, and disaster care, may be lead by a nurse and/or physician coordinator for pediatric emergency care.[1]

In addition to employees and other hospital-based clinical staff, hospital planning should consider available clinical resources in the community. Pre-authorization of clinical and non-clinical disaster volunteers is a measure that can be taken to avoid the chaos that may result when well-intended volunteers respond to facilities during a disaster. One way to limit this chaos is to identify community support systems prior to needing them, and to incorporate the support of local pediatricians and family practitioners who are willing to assist with pediatric care in the event of a major disaster. Medical volunteers with pediatric experience can be identified in advance, and their professional credentialing information maintained in a hospital data base.[61] Including individuals that can assist with the care of children, particularly children with special health care needs, is vital as the hospital may not have sufficient personnel with specialized pediatric care skills to care for children in all care settings (emergency department, ambulatory care, inpatient care, critical care, etc.). Hospitals should also consider state and federal disaster response teams as a potential resource, and work with those entities proactively toward the development of pediatric readiness.

A predetermined disaster staffing model can assist organizations and communities as they develop their pediatric disaster plans. A core group of dedicated pediatric staff that are able to "ride out" the acute event should be established with a secondary group prepared to provide relief. All staff should be well educated and trained in pediatric disaster care and be able to function in their proposed role in a disaster before it occurs. Having such training reinforced as part of an annual pediatric mass-casualty drill, and monitoring via regular assessments of core clinical competencies, will be useful in maintaining readiness.[60] The institution should also have a plan to help staff members care for their own family members during a time of crisis. This may include setting up an on-site family care center.[62]

In summary, the ED functions as the "front door" to the hospital organization, and as a primary interface between the hospital and the community it serves. Emergency departments must foster an environment of care that emphasizes pediatric patient safety and care quality. This commitment to quality and safety must be maintained during disaster events. A hospital's preparedness for a pediatric mass-casualty event should be built upon a strong foundation of day-to-day readiness for pediatric emergencies. Efforts to promote and maintain pediatric readiness should be lead by a nurse and/or physician

---

TABLE 8-1

Pediatric Issues in Disaster Shelter Planning Supplies and Services

- Access to telephone consultation for medical questions
- Basic pediatric first-aid equipment and guidelines
- Child-appropriate nutrition
- Diapers and other supplies for infant hygiene
- Games and other distractions for children
- Infant formula and rehydration solutions

Staffing
- Prepare staff members to help supervise children when parents start recovery efforts.
- Set contingencies so that the entire family of a child with special health care needs can be together.
- Train staff members in basic pediatric emergency care.
- Use family volunteers to help supervise children.

Safety
- Childproof the shelter to promote safety for children and the elderly.
- Sequester sick children and their families to reduce the spread of illness.
- Set ground rules for a healthy environment (limit or forbid smoking, drinking, weapons).
- Supervise interactions between children and frail (often elderly) shelter occupants.

Source: Romig L.: Disaster management. In Gausche-Hill M., Fuchs S., Yamamoto L. (eds.): APLS: *The Pediatric Emergency Medicine Resource,* Revised 4th ed. Sudbury, MA: Jones and Bartlett, 2007. Printed with permission.

---

coordinator for pediatric emergency care. Ultimately, support from multiple hospital departments and community- and hospital-based professionals will be required to assure pediatric emergency and disaster preparedness. All aspects of a hospital's disaster plan should include considerations for children and families, and these plans should be regularly tested to assure optimal readiness.

References

1. Gausche-Hill M., Krug S., and the American Academy of Pediatrics Committee on Pediatric Emergency Medicine, American College of Emergency Physicians Pediatric Committee, and the Emergency Nurses Association: Guidelines for the care of children in the emergency department. *Pediatrics* 2009.

2. Romig L.: Disaster management. In Gausche-Hill M., Fuchs S., Yamamoto L. (eds.): APLS: *The Pediatric Emergency Medicine Resource,* 4th ed. Sudbury, MA: Jones and Bartlett, 2004.

3. Foltin G.L., Schonfeld D.J., Shannon M. (eds.): Pediatric terrorism and disaster preparedness: a resource for pediatricians. Rockville, MD: Agency for Healthcare Research and Quality, 2006. Available at: http://www.ahrq.gov/RESEARCH/PEDPREP/resource.htm (accessed Mar. 1, 2009).

4. American Academy of Pediatrics Committee on Pediatric Emergency Medicine Committee on Medical Liability and the Task Force on Terrorism: The pediatrician and disaster preparedness. *Pediatrics* 117(2):560–565, 2006.

5. Markenson D., Reynolds S., AAP Committee on Pediatric Emergency Medicine and Task Force on Terrorism: The pediatrician and disaster preparedness: technical report. *Pediatrics* 117(2):e340–362, 2006.

6. Dolan M.A., Krug S.E.: Pediatric disaster preparedness in the wake of Katrina: lessons to be learned. *Clin Pediatr Emerg Med* 7(1):59–66, 2006.

7. Foltin G., Knapp J.: How are children different. In Foltin G., Tunik M., Treiber M., Cooper A. (eds.): *Pediatric disaster preparedness: a resource for planning, management and provision of out-of-hospital emergency care.* New York, NY: Center for Pediatric Emergency Medicine, 2008.

8. Henretig F., McKee M.R.: Preparedness for acts of nuclear, biological and chemical terrorism. In Gausche-Hill M., Fuchs S., Yamamoto L. (eds.): APLS: *The Pediatric Emergency Medicine Resource,* 4th ed. Sudbury, MA: Jones and Bartlett, 2004.

9. Henretig F.M., Cieslak T.J., Eitzen E.M.: Biological and chemical terrorism. *J Pediatr* 141(3):311–326, 2002.

10. Lovejoy J.C. Initial approach to patient management after large scale disasters. *Clin Pediatr Emerg Med* 3:217–223, 2002.

11. Shenoi R. Chemical warfare agents. *Clin Pediatr Emerg Med* 3:239–247, 2002.

12. American Academy of Pediatrics Committee on Environmental Health and Committee on Infectious Diseases: Chemical-biological terrorism and its impact upon children. *Pediatrics* 118(3):1276–1287, 2006.

13. Allen J.T., Matthews L.M.: Radiation as a weapon of mass destruction. *Clin Pediatr Emerg Med* 3:248–255, 2002.

14. American Academy of Pediatrics Committee on Environmental Health: Radiation disasters and children. *Pediatrics* 111(6):1455–1466, 2003.

15. Shannon M., Chung S.: Topical decontamination of children. In Foltin G., Tunik M., Treiber M., Cooper A. (eds.): *Pediatric disaster preparedness: a resource for planning, management and provision of out-of-hospital emergency care.* New York, NY: Center for Pediatric Emergency Medicine, 2008.

16. Dieckmann R.A.: Pediatric assessment. In Gausche-Hill M., Fuchs S., Yamamoto L. (eds.): APLS: *The Pediatric Emergency Medicine Resource,* 4th ed. Sudbury, MA: Jones and Bartlett, 2004.

17. Ralston M., Hazinski M.F., Zaritsky A.L., et al. (eds.): American Heart Association and American Academy of Pediatrics: PALS course guide and PALS provider manual: provider manual. Dallas, TX: American Heart Association, 2007.

18. Maxon R.T.: Management of pediatric trauma: blast victims in a mass casualty incident. *Clin Pediatr Emerg Med* 3:256–261, 2002.

19. Tuggle D., Krug S., American Academy of Pediatrics Section on Orthopaedics, Committee on Pediatric Emergency Medicine, Section on Critical Care, Section on Surgery, Section on Transport Medicine, Committee on Pediatric Emergency Medicine, Pediatric Orthopaedic Society Of North America: Management of pediatric trauma. *Pediatrics* 121(4):849–854, 2008.

20. Tepas J.J., Fallat M.E., Moriarty T.M.: Trauma. In Gausche-Hill M., Fuchs S., Yamamoto L. (eds.): APLS: *The Pediatric Emergency Medicine Resource,* 4th ed. Sudbury, MA: Jones and Bartlett, 2004.

21. Hagan J.F., AAP Committee on Psychosocial Aspects of Child and Family Health and the Task Force on Terrorism: Psychosocial implications of disaster or terrorism on children: a guide for the pediatrician. *Pediatrics* 116(3):787–795, 2005.

22. Schonfeld D.: Psychological first aid. In Foltin G., Tunik M., Treiber M., Cooper A. (eds.): *Pediatric disaster preparedness: a resource for planning, management and provision of out-of-hospital emergency care.* New York, NY: Center for Pediatric Emergency Medicine, 2008.

23. Magrid P.A., Grant R., Reilly M.J., Redlener N.B.: Short-term impact of a major disaster on children's mental health: building resiliency in the aftermath of Hurricane Katrina. *Pediatrics* 117(5)S448–453, 2006.

24. Smitherman H., Soloway-Simon D.: Special needs of children following a disaster. *Clin Pediatr Emerg Med* 3(4):262–267, 2002.

25. Treadwell-Deering D., Hanisch S.: Psychological response to disaster in children and families. *Clin Pediatr Emerg Med* 3(4):268–274, 2002.

26. Fairbrother G., Stuber J., Galea S., et al.: Unmet need for counseling services by children in New York City after the September 11th attacks on the World Trade Center: implications for pediatricians. *Pediatrics* 113(5):1367–1374, 2004.

27. Ziegler M.F., Greenwald M.H., DeGuzman M.A., Simon H.K. Posttraumatic stress responses in children: awareness and practice among a sample of pediatric emergency care providers. *Pediatrics* 115(5):1261–1267, 2005.

28. Broughton D.D., Allen J.D., Hannemann R.E., Petrikin J.E.: Reuniting fractured families after a disaster: the role of the National Center for Missing and Exploited Children. *Pediatrics* 117(5):S442–445, 2006.

29. Maxin C.: Patient identification and tracking. In Foltin G., Tunik M., Treiber M., Cooper A. (eds.): *Pediatric disaster preparedness: a resource for planning, management and provision of out-of-hospital emergency care.* New York, NY: Center for Pediatric Emergency Medicine, 2008.

30. Chung S., Shannon M.: Reuniting children with their families during disasters: a proposed plan for greater success. *Am J Disaster Med* 2:113–117, 2007.

31. Pediatric security issues during a disaster. Pediatric disaster toolkit: Hospital guidelines for pediatrics during disasters, 2nd ed., 2006. New York City Department of Health and Mental Hygiene. Available at: http://www.nyc.gov/html/doh/downloads/word/bhpp/bhpp-focus-ped-toolkit-1-security.doc (accessed Mar. 1, 2009).

32. Save the Children Federation: Safe spaces: a signature program. Available at: http://www.savethechildren.org/programs/us-literacy-and-nutrition/safe-spaces-us.html (accessed Mar. 1, 2009).

33. Distephano S.M., Graf J.M., Lowry A.W., Sitler G.C. Preparing, improvising, and caring for children during mass transport after a disaster. *Pediatrics* 117(5):S421–427, 2006.

34. Family information and support center: Pediatric disaster toolkit: Hospital guidelines for pediatrics during disasters, 2nd ed., 2006. New York City Department of Health and Mental Hygiene. Available at: http://www.nyc.gov/html/doh/downloads/word/bhpp/bhpp-focus-ped-toolkit-13-family.doc (accessed Mar. 1, 2009).

35. Tunik M.: Children with special health care needs. In Foltin G., Tunik M., Treiber M., Cooper A. (eds.): *Pediatric disaster preparedness: a resource for planning, management and provision of out-of-hospital emergency care.* New York, NY: Center for Pediatric Emergency Medicine, 2008.

36. Greenwald P.W., Rutherford A.F., Green R.A., Giglio J.: Emergency department visits for home medical device failure during the 2003 North America blackout. *Acad Emerg Med* 11(7):786–789, 2004.

37. Klein K.R., Rosenthal M.S., Klausner H.A.: Blackout 2003: lessons learned from the perspectives of four hospitals. *Prehosp Disast Med* 20(5):343–349, 2005.

38. Arquilla B., Treiber M.: Disaster drills. In Foltin G., Tunik M., Treiber M., Cooper A. (eds.): *Pediatric disaster preparedness: a resource for planning, management and provision of out-of-hospital emergency care.* New York, NY: Center for Pediatric Emergency Medicine, 2008.

39. Weiner D., Manzi S., Waltzman M., et al.: The natural disaster medical system response: a pediatric perspective. *Pediatrics* 117(5):S405–411, 2006.

40. Institute of Medicine, Committee on the Future of Emergency Care in the United States Health System: Emergency care for children: growing pains. Washington, D.C.: National Academies Press, 2006.

41. Shirm S., Liggin R., Dick R., Graham J.: Prehospital preparedness for pediatric mass-casualty events. *Pediatrics* 120:e756–761, 2007.

42. Graham J., Shirm S., Jiggin R., et al.: Mass-casualty events at schools: a national preparedness survey. *Pediatrics* 117(1):e8–15, 2006.

43. Wan R.P., Olympia E., Avner J.R. The preparedness of schools to respond to children in emergencies: a national survey of school nurses. *Pediatrics* 116(6):e736–749, 2005.

44. Sirbaugh P.E., Gurwitch K.D., Macias C.G., et al.: Creation and implementation of a mobile pediatric emergency response team: regionalized caring for displaced children after a disaster. *Pediatrics* 117(5):S428–438, 2006.

45. Sirbaugh P.: Urgent care. In Foltin G., Tunik M., Treiber M., Cooper A. (eds.): *Pediatric disaster preparedness: a resource for planning, management and provision of out-of-hospital emergency care.* New York, NY: Center for Pediatric Emergency Medicine, 2008.

46. Allen G.M., Parrillo S., Will J., Mohr J.A.: Principles of disaster planning for the pediatric population. *Prehosp Disast Med* 22(6):537–540, 2007.

47. Emergency Medical Services for Children: Strategic plan FY 2008– FY 2010. Recommendations of the partnership for children stakeholder's group. Washington, D.C.: EMSC National Resource Center. Available at: http://www.childrensnational.org/files/PDF/EMSC/PubRes/Public_Version_of_Final_EMSC_Strategic_Plan.pdf (accessed Mar. 1, 2009).

48. National Center for Disaster Preparedness: Pediatric preparedness for disasters and terrorism. National consensus conference. Columbia University Mailman School of Public Health, March 2007. Available at: http://www.ncdp.mailman.columbia.edu/files/peds2.pdf (accessed Mar. 1, 2009).

49. Romig L.: Pediatric triage on-scene in disasters. In Foltin G., Tunik M., Treiber M., Cooper A. (eds.): *Pediatric disaster preparedness: a resource for planning, management and provision of out-of-hospital emergency care.* New York, NY: Center for Pediatric Emergency Medicine, 2008.

50. Pediatric hospital-based disaster triage. Pediatric disaster toolkit: Hospital guidelines for pediatrics during disasters, 2nd ed., 2006. New York City Department of Health and Mental Hygiene. Available at: http://www.nyc.gov/html/doh/downloads/word/bhpp/bhpp-focus-ped-toolkit-12-triage.doc (accessed Mar. 1, 2009).

51. START: Simple triage and rapid treatment. Critical illness and trauma foundation. Available at: http://www.citmt.org/start/default.htm (accessed Mar. 1, 2009).

52. Romig L.E.: Pediatric triage. A system to JumpSTART your triage of young patients at MCIs. *J Emerg Med Serv* 27(7):52–8, 60–63, 2002.

53. Vayer J.S., Ten Eyck R.P., Cowan M.L.: New triage concepts in triage. *Ann Emerg Med;* 15(8):927–930, 1986.

54. Fendya D.: When disaster strikes: care considerations for pediatric patients. *J Trauma Nurs* 13(4):161–165, 2006.

55. Shannon M., Chung S.: Topical decontamination of children. In Foltin G., Tunik M., Treiber M., Cooper A. (eds.): *Pediatric disaster preparedness: a resource for planning, management and provision of out-of-hospital emergency care.* New York, NY: Center for Pediatric Emergency Medicine, 2008.

56. Scalzo A., Lehman-Huskamp K.L., Sinks G.A., Keenan W.J.: Disaster preparedness and toxic exposures in children. *Clin Pediatr Emerg Med* 9:47–60, 2008.

57. Pediatric decontamination. Pediatric disaster toolkit: Hospital guidelines for pediatrics during disasters, 2nd ed., 2006. New York City Department of Health and Mental Hygiene. Available at: http://www.nyc.gov/html/doh/downloads/word/bhpp/bhpp-focus-ped-toolkit-8-decon.doc (accessed Mar. 1, 2009).

58. Surge considerations. Pediatric disaster toolkit: Hospital guidelines for pediatrics during disasters, 2nd ed., 2006. New York City Department of Health and Mental Hygiene. Available at: http://www.nyc.gov/html/doh/downloads/word/bhpp/bhpp-focus-ped-toolkit-3-surge.doc (accessed Mar. 1, 2009).

59. Bradley R.: Shelter care. In Foltin G., Tunik M., Treiber M., Cooper A. (eds.): *Pediatric disaster preparedness: a resource for planning, management and provision of out-of-hospital emergency care.* New York, NY: Center for Pediatric Emergency Medicine, 2008.

60. Staffing recommendations for pediatrics during a disaster. Pediatric disaster toolkit: Hospital guidelines for pediatrics during disasters, 2nd ed., 2006. New York City Department of Health and Mental Hygiene. Available at: http://www.nyc.gov/html/doh/downloads/word/bhpp/bhpp-focus-ped-toolkit-7-staffing.doc (accessed Mar. 1, 2009).

61. Brown O.W.: Hurricane Katrina experiences: receiving patients in Longview, Texas, 350 miles from ground zero. *Pediatrics* 117(5):S439–441, 2006.

62. Buttross S.: Caring for the children of caretakers during a disaster. *Pediatrics* 117(5):S446–447, 2006.

List of Abbreviations

AAP	American Academy of Pediatrics
ACEP	American College of Emergency Physicians
ADM	automated dispensing machine
AFB	acid-fast bacilli
AHA	American Heart Association
APLS	Advanced Pediatric Life Support
ASA	American Society of Anesthesiologists
BATHE	Background; Affect; Trouble; Handling; Empathy
B-SAFER	Bio-Surveillance Analysis, Feedback, Evaluation, and Response
CDC	Centers for Disease Control and Prevention
CPEN	certified pediatric emergency nurse
CPOE	computerized physician order entry
CRM	Crew Resource Management
CT	computerized tomography
DMAT	Disaster Medical Assistance Team
ED	emergency department
EIF	emergency information form
EMR	electronic medical record
EMS	Emergency Medical Services
EMSC	Emergency Medical Services for Children
ENA	Emergency Nurses Association
ENPC	Emergency Nursing Pediatric Care
ESBL	extended spectrum beta-lactamases
FMEA	failure mode effects analysis
HBIG	hepatitis B immune globulin
IOM	Institute of Medicine
JCR	Joint Commission Resources
LASA	Look-Alike and Sound-Alike
LILY	Lifesaving Interventions for Little Youth

LIP	Licensed Independent Practitioner
MDRO	Multidrug-resistant organism
MEMSCIS	Minnesota Emergency Medical Services for Children Information System
MRSA	methicillin-resistant *Staphylococcus aureus*
NPSG	National Patient Safety Goal
PALS	Pediatric Advanced Life Support
PAT	Pediatric Assessment Triangle
PCA	patient-controlled analgesia
PCP	primary care provider
PEP	post-exposure prophylaxis
PEPP	Pediatric Education for Prehospital Professionals
PFCC	patient- and family-centered care
PI	performance improvement
PPE	personal protective equipment
QI	quality improvement
RFI	requirement for improvement
RIG	rabies immune globulin
RN	registered nurse
RODS	Real-time Outbreak and Disease Surveillance
RSV	respiratory syncytial virus
SARS	severe acute respiratory syndrome
SBAR	Situation-Background-Assessment-Recommendation
SCOPE	Special Children's Outreach and Prehospital Education
START	Simple Triage and Rapid Treatment
SSTI	skin and soft tissue infection
TDaP	acellular pertussis vaccine component
VRE	vancomycin-resistant enterococci

Index

Note: Page numbers followed by *f* and *t* indicate figures and tables respectively.

A

AAP. *See* American Academy of Pediatrics (AAP)

Abbreviations, in medication prescribing, 57

Abdominal pain, causes in pediatric population, 98, 101, 102*t*

Abduction

    measures preventing, 48–49

    tabletop drill, 49

Abscess, incision and drainage of, PPE recommendations for, 79*t*

Accident causation, "Swiss Cheese" model of, 6, 6*f*

ACEP. *See* American College of Emergency Physicians (ACEP)

Adenovirus, diarrhea and, contact precautions for, 78

ADMs (automated dispensing machines), 56, 61, 69

Adolescents

    abdominal pain causes in, 102*t*

    age definition for, 96

    depressive signs and symptoms in, 111*t*, 112

    interviews with, 36

Adults, pediatric patients and

    differences between, 97, 99*t*–100*t*

        in disaster situation, 130–132

    medical imaging risks, 105

Advanced Pediatric Life Support (APLS), 126

Adverse drug events

    dosage calculations, 59

    factors contributing to, 60

    incidence of, 53–54

    interruptions causing, 59

    occurrence rates, 54

    prescribing errors

        avoiding, 57

        types, 63, 69–70

Adverse patient events, 3–4

Age, behavioral characteristics and, 97–98, 101*t*

Age-based vital signs, 96–97, 98*t*

Agency for Healthcare Research and Quality (AHRQ), 28

Airborne-transmission precautions, 77, 77*t*

ALARA (as low as reasonably achievable), radiation exposure, 105–106

Alcohol-based solutions. *See* Waterless antiseptic agents

Allergy, to medication, 56

Alliance for Radiation Safety in Pediatric Imaging, 106

Amber Alerts, 49

American Academy of Pediatrics (AAP)

    clinical competency recommendations, 96, 97, 138

    emergency care

        care plan recommendations for, 122

        guidelines for, ix, 6, 9, 11

            providing information for, 118–119, 120*t*–121*t*

        for trauma, recommendations, 107

    pediatric care standards, 17

    sedation guidelines, 71, 72–73

American College of Emergency Physicians (ACEP)

    emergency information form, 118–119, 120*t*–121*t*

    emergency pediatric care guidelines, ix, 6, 9, 11

    pediatric care standards, 17

    pediatric clinical competency recommendations, 96, 97, 138

Analgesia/sedation, monitoring and managing, 70–71

    AAP guidelines, 71, 72–73

Anatomical differences, between adult and pediatric populations, 99*t*

    in disaster situation, 130

Anthrax exposure, 87*t*

Antibiotics, broad-spectrum, 103

Antiretroviral prophylaxis, post-exposure, 89

Antiseptic agents, waterless, 76

Antiviral chemoprophylaxis, in pandemic influenza, 83